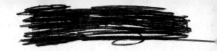

HELPING CHILDREN COPE
WITH STAMMERING

TRUDY STEWART & JACKIE TURNBULL are experienced speech and language therapists based in Leeds. They specialise in working with children and adults who stammer and have written numerous articles and a book for professionals, *Working with Dysfluent Children*, published in 1995 by Winslow Press.

They are actively involved in the British Stammering Association and generally in promoting the needs of their clients in schools and the work place. They believe the best outcomes are achieved by working in partnership with their clients, families and others to help them achieve their potential.

Overcoming Common Problems Series

For a full list of titles please contact
Sheldon Press, Marylebone Road, London NW1 4DU

The Assertiveness Workbook
A plan for busy women
JOANNA CUTMANN

Beating the Comfort Trap
DR WINDY DRYDEN AND JACK
GORDON

Birth Over Thirty Five
SHEILA KITZINGER

Body Language
How to read others' thoughts by their
gestures
ALLAN PEASE

Body Language in Relationships
DAVID COHEN

Calm Down
How to cope with frustration and anger
DR PAUL HAUCK

Cancer – A Family Affair
NEVILLE SHONE

Comfort for Depression
JANET HORWOOD

Coping Successfully with Hayfever
DR ROBERT YOUNGSON

Coping Successfully with Migraine
SUE DYSON

Coping Successfully with Pain
NEVILLE SHONE

Coping Successfully with PMS
KAREN EVENNETT

Coping Successfully with Panic Attacks
SHIRLEY TRICKETT

**Coping Successfully with Prostrate
Problems**
ROSY REYNOLDS

**Coping Successfully with Your
Hyperactive Child**
DR PAUL CARSON

**Coping Successfully with Your Irritable
Bowel**
ROSEMARY NICOL

**Coping Successfully with Your Second
Child**
FIONA MARSHALL

Coping with Anxiety and Depression
SHIRLEY TRICKETT

Coping with Blushing
DR ROBERT EDELMANN

Coping with Bronchitis and Emphysema
DR TOM SMITH

Coping with Candida
SHIRLEY TRICKETT

Coping with Chronic Fatigue
TRUDIE CHALDER

Coping with Cot Death
SARAH MURPHY

Coping with Crushes
ANITA NAIK

Coping with Cystitis
CAROLINE CLAYTON

Coping with Depression and Elation
DR PATRICK McKEON

Coping with Postnatal Depression
FIONA MARSHALL

Coping with Psoriasis
PROFESSOR RONALD MARKS

Coping with Schizophrenia
DR STEVEN JONES AND DR FRANK
TALLIS

Coping with Strokes
DR TOM SMITH

Coping with Suicide
DR DONALD SCOTT

Coping with Thyroid Problems
DR JOAN GOMEZ

Coping with Thrush
CAROLINE CLAYTON

Curing Arthritis Exercise Book
MARGARET HILLS AND JANET
HORWOOD

Curing Arthritis Diet Book
MARGARET HILLS

Curing Arthritis – The Drug-Free Way
MARGARET HILLS

Overcoming Common Problems Series

Curing Arthritis
More ways to a drug-free life
MARGARET HILLS

Curing Illness – The Drug-Free Way
MARGARET HILLS

Depression
DR PAUL HAUCK

Divorce and Separation
Every woman's guide to a new life
ANGELA WILLANS

Don't Blame Me!
How to stop blaming yourself and other people
TONY GOUGH

Everything Parents Should Know About Drugs
SARAH LAWSON

Family First Aid and Emergency Handbook
DR ANDREW STANWAY

Getting Along with People
DIANNE DOUBTFIRE

Getting the Best for Your Bad Back
DR ANYTHONY CAMPBELL

Good Stress Guide, The
MARY HARTLEY

Heart Attacks – Prevent and Survive
DR TOM SMITH

Helping Children Cope with Bullying
SARAH LAWSON

Helping Children Cope with Divorce
ROSEMARY WELLS

Helping Children Cope with Grief
ROSEMARY WELLS

Hold Your Head Up High
DR PAUL HAUCK

How to Be Your Own Best Friend
DR PAUL HAUCK

How to Cope when the Going Gets Tough
DR WINDY DRYDEN AND JACK GORDON

How to Cope with Bulimia
DR JOAN GOMEZ

How to Cope with Difficult People
ALAN HOUEL WITH CHRISTIAN GODEFROY

How to Cope with Splitting Up
VERA PEIFFER

How to Cope with Stress
DR PETER TYRER

How to Cope with your Child's Allergies
DR PAUL CARSON

How to Do What You Want to Do
DR PAUL HAUCK

How to Improve Your Confidence
DR KENNETH HAMBLY

How to Interview and Be Interviewed
MICHELE BROWN AND GYLES BRANDRETH

How to Keep Your Cholesterol in Check
DR ROBERT POVEY

How to Love and Be Loved
DR PDAUL HAUCK

How to Pass Your Driving Test
DONALD RIDLAND

How to Stand up for Yourself
DR PAUL HAUCK

How to Start a Conversation and Make Friends
DON GABOR

How to Stop Smoking
GEORGE TARGET

How to Stop Worrying
DR FRANK TALLIS

How to Survive Your Teenagers
SHEILA DAINOW

How to Untangle Your Emotional Knots
DR WINDY DRYDEN AND JACK GORDON

How to Write a Successful CV
JOANNA GUTMANN

Hysterectomy
SUZIE HAYMAN

Is HRT Right for You?
DR ANNE MACGREGOR

The Incredible Sulk
DR WINDY DRYDEN

The Irritable Bowel Diet Book
ROSEMARY NICOL

The Irritable Bowel Stress Book
ROSEMARY NICOL

Overcoming Common Problems Series

Overcoming Common Problems

HELPING CHILDREN COPE
WITH STAMMERING

Jackie Turnbull
and Trudy Stewart

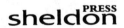

First published in Great Britain in 1996 by
Sheldon Press, SPCK, Marylebone Road, London NW1 4DU

British Library Cataloguing-in-Publication Data
A catalogue record for this book is available from the British Library

ISBN 0–85969–728–2

Photoset by Deltatype Ltd, Ellesmere Port, Cheshire
Printed in Great Britain by J.W. Arrowsmith Ltd., Bristol

For all the non-fluent children and their carers we have met in our clinics. They have taught us much about this difficulty and its impact on their lives, which is so often underestimated and misunderstood.

Contents

Acknowledgements

With thanks to our friends and colleagues, Lesley Hodgkinson, Juliette Gregory, Monica Bray and for their tolerance innovative ideas, committment and personal support.

Introduction

When we first entered the world of Speech and Language Therapy, we were both immediately drawn to the area of dysfluency. We found it fascinating in so many ways and unlike many of the other speech problems we had been trained to deal with. There were, and still are, far more questions than answers. We puzzled, for example, over such issues as why most children who stammered were in fact fluent most of the time; why fluency levels could vary so dramatically in the same child from one word or sentence or day to the next; why some children very quickly became upset about relatively mild dysfluency and others seemed oblivious of dysfluency which to the listener seemed much more severe.

In our early days of working with people who stammer, we wondered whether we might one day write a book on the subject. We even pondered over the title. In our imagination we called it 'It's a funny thing, stammering'. By this, of course, we did not mean 'funny ha-ha', because we already knew something of the anguish which stammering could cause. Rather we meant 'funny peculiar', because the problem seemed such a difficult one to get to grips with or even to say anything certain about. Indeed, 20 years on, we still have no definitive answers to all those questions we are asked or have asked ourselves about such important and fundamental areas as 'what causes stammering, what maintains it, what makes it go away?'. This lack of knowledge, whilst frustrating at times, also drives us on to find out more and to seek new approaches to helping people who stammer – both to maximize their potential fluency but more importantly to live lives which are affected as little as possible by their lack of speech fluency.

This particular book (with a revised title!) has come about for a number of reasons. It has developed from our contact with our own clients and from a desire to be able to offer some reading to supplement our face to face work with them. Many parents are eager to read as much as they can in order to understand dysfluency and thus help their children. However, when they go to bookshops or libraries they discover that there is very little available. Most of the books are written for professionals and not for carers. Consequently they are full of technical jargon and may be difficult for those outside of the speech and language therapy profession to understand. Some books written for non-professionals seem to us to be too dogmatic; they are full of do's and don'ts and appear not to consider the individual nature of children and their carers. Consequently carers often end up feeling more guilty when they have read them, and more of a failure if they are unable to live up to the high standards which are set. (We know this because we sometimes have to pick up the pieces in our clinics!) We hope this book fills that gap. We hope too that it will provide something rather different from those books which *are* currently available, for a number of reasons. Firstly, it is written mainly for parents and carers using lay peoples' terms and where more technical terms are employed, they are explained. Secondly, it deals exclusively with children and young people. Thirdly, it is intended to be a practical book, aimed at helping parents to cope more effectively and resourcefully with both their feelings about and their behaviour towards their dysfluent children.

Our desire to write this book also came from our work with adults who stammer. For many of them, the problems they currently face are rooted in their childhood experiences. The following example illustrates what we mean. A man who stammers queues at a self-service restaurant. He feels the tension building up inside as he decides whether to choose chilli con carne (which he wants but fears he cannot say fluently) or go instead for an egg salad (which he does not want but feels he *can* say fluently). So often we are told it is at this point that he feels he is back in childhood. He is flooded with memories of an incident where he faced the same agonizing decisions and where his worst fears were borne out – perhaps he asked for a beefburger, stammered badly and felt humiliated, embarrassed, ashamed and much more. Our adult clients often tell us that they wish they had been able to talk about events such as these with a friend or sympathetic adult, that their school could have been more aware of the difficulties they were experiencing and that they had been given some strategies for coping. They wish they could have received more help from their parents, but their parents felt at a loss. They may have received conflicting advice: been told, for example, to ignore it by some people and correct it by others. We hope this book will help today's parents provide some real help and understanding. Then, even if their worst fears are realized and their child stammers into adulthood, the young person can still feel good about himself and his communication and say the things he really wants to.

Most importantly, the book has developed from our own beliefs about stammering. As we will see in the early chapters, there are many (often conflicting) ideas about the cause and nature of stammering, and thus we are not able to offer the reader very much in the way of concrete facts. However, are able to share our current knowledge about stammering and to outline ideas regarding the help parents can give, as well as explain the professional help available. What we offer stems from a twofold premise in which we believe and on which our therapy is based. The first belief is that parents do not cause stammering. The second is that they can help their children manage it more effectively and minimize the harmful effects that having a stammer may bring. In this book we aim to look at ways in which this may be done.

Finally in this section, we thought readers might like to know a little about our own work with dysfluent clients. We have both worked in this field for many years and in 1978 began to run groups together for adults who stammer. Currently we work with dysfluent clients of all ages, individually, in families and in intensive and non-intensive groups. We also have involvement with the wider community. Our regular visits to schools, involve both discussion of individual children and also education of others as to the nature of stammering and the part they can play in helping their dysfluent classmates. We work with relatives of people who stammer and sometimes have contact with their workplaces. Another area which we see as important is the sharing of our thoughts with others: we regularly lecture on stammering and also attend courses and seminars to update ourselves on current practice in our own and other professions. We try to be as open-minded as possible about our therapy – to realize that different approaches are needed for different people and that new ideas are continually being thought of all the time which we need to look at carefully before accepting or rejecting. We believe we are especially fortunate to have built up a good personal and professional relationship over the many years we have known each other and to be able to use each other as sounding boards to develop our ideas.

1

What is stammering?

Why are you reading this book?

You have probably been attracted to this book because you know someone with a stammer, perhaps you have a friend who stammers, maybe you have heard someone in your immediate family stammering, it could be your own child, it may even be you. Lots of people experience stammering-type speech at least sometime in their lives. However, the fact that it is more common than we think does not seem to make much difference. Stammering is worrying – it can be difficult to listen to and is not easy to live with on a daily basis.

Defining stammering

But what is this type of talking that we all call stammering? Well, there is our first problem – not everyone calls it stammering. The Americans refer to the same mode of speech as stuttering. The term is sometimes used in Britain, but usually stammering is the accepted label. Nevertheless stammering and stuttering mean exactly the same thing. Back to the question – what do we mean when we talk about stammering? It seems to be something that we know about almost instinctively. If we hear someone in the bank or post office speaking in a certain way, a little light goes on in our heads and we think 'He's got a stammer'. Interestingly we rarely respond similarly if we hear a child with a croaky voice or a toddler having difficulty saying a particular sound, like 's' or 'r'. So as speakers ourselves we can (or think we can) identify stammering and stammerers fairly easily when we listen to others. Frequently we describe what we hear as 'blocking' or 'hesitancy' in speech, and we may describe the person themselves as nervous, anxious, lacking in self-confidence, although, as we shall see later, this is rarely true.

We are not born with an innate ability to label stammering. It appears to be something we learn to do, acquiring our knowledge from others or from society at large. Children, especially young children, do not share the same perception as we adults. This was well illustrated when a young client visiting our clinic was asked what she did when she got stuck on a word. She replied, 'Oh, I just go and ask my mum what the word says'. This showed us that for her 'getting stuck' only happened when she read and she was unsure of a word. As an adult we might have labelled some

5

parts of her talking as stammering, but she did not think of it in the same way and limited her labelling to her reading speech.

However, some children do learn to view it in our adult way. They develop their own labels for it and we see them often struggling to make sense of it. Some children we have met have talked about a loss of control or a need to wait before they can begin to speak. It is as if their speech muscles act independently and cannot be easily directed. 'It is when your words get stuck' is a common interpretation. Looking at this definition we can see the child has an awareness that the words he wished to say were there, formed in his head, but somehow the route to the outside world was impeded.

Obvious stammering

Speech and language therapists talk about stammering in terms of a loss of the fluency of speech. This is different from the popular sense of the word fluency, in which language is perceived as a continuous stream of interesting words spoken with apparent ease and speed. For the therapist, stammering or *dys*fluency, a word we will use throughout this book, refers to a problem resulting from a disruption in the flow and timing of speech. This disruption can take a number of different forms, and we list the main ones below.

Repetition A particular part of speech may be repeated a number of times, such as a word, as in 'That man, man, man's got a hat, hat on'. Other parts of speech such as sounds and phrases can also be repeated, as in 'Where is my, where is my b-b-ball, Mummy?' These repetitions may be spoken in an easy, quite slow way or can be produced in quick succession, sounding like rapid gun fire. As we shall see later this difference can be significant.

Prolongation Sounds may be produced with added length, as in 'I f—eel s—ick'. This prolongation of sound can be produced in a relaxed manner or may be filled with tension as if the child is pushing the sound out of his mouth. Once again this difference is an important one to consider.

Hesitation There may be pauses in the child's speech. These hesitations often occur at the beginning of an utterance and the listener may notice the child trying hard to get started into what they want to say. There may also be gaps between words which do not follow the sense of the sentence. For example, 'I like watching – cartoons on – telly'. In some children you have a feeling that this is because the child does not know the right word to say and is in the process of searching around in his head in an attempt to find it. Alternatively when you listen to other children you sense they know the word they wish to say and the struggle is actually in getting that word out. Finally, pauses can occur in the middle of words, such as 'Someti.– mes my bro – ther is a pest'.

Freezing In some instances a child seems to freeze before saying a sound or word or even in the middle of saying it. It is as though a clock has stopped and his speech muscles are frozen in time and space until the magic moment when someone or something clicks and the suspended animation is released.

Fillers Extra words or sounds may be added which do not contribute to the meaning of the speech, as in 'I, you know, like, you know, jaffa cakes best' or 'I, ermm, like, ermm, jaffa cakes best'.

Forcing A child can be heard to push some sounds out in a forceful way. It is as if the mechanism is jammed and with a little extra effort the flow can be resumed.

Incompletion Sometimes words and/or sentences may be left unfinished.

Airflow problems Breathing may be disrupted; the child can feel as if he does not have enough air to finish his sentences or perhaps he takes lots of short gasps of air.

Gestures In some cases extra movements of the face and/or body become associated with the child's attempts to talk. She blinks her eyes or stamps her foot in frustration one day and somehow she finds she can get the word out. This is then repeated the next time she gets stuck on a word and so a pattern is established.

Eye contact Sometimes a child is unable to look at his listener. A child may break the communication link, loose eye contact and look away at times when he perceives that his speech is running into difficulties, when he thinks he is losing control or is fearful that at any moment he might. It can be this very act of looking away which draws the listener's attention to the fact that something is wrong. This is very often the opposite result the child had hoped for – by looking away he had hoped to conceal his difficulties.

Hidden stammering

All these examples above are types of behaviours which we as listeners are able to identify because we can see and hear them. However, there are types of stammering which are not so readily observable but

7

nevertheless are part of the stammering armoury. These hidden aspects of stammering relate to the thoughts and feelings which a stammering child has.

Speech avoidance A child may avoid saying a sound or word which he thinks is difficult to say. He may change the word in his head and substitute another with a similar meaning. Whole sentences can be changed around to avoid having to say a word in a certain context. Perhaps worst of all the child opts out of talking altogether: he may ask a friend to do his talking for him, pretend he does not know what to say, has forgotten or does not know the answer to a question. It is better that other children, teachers and family think he is less intelligent, less verbal, less sociable than think he is a stammerer.

Situation avoidance Another type of avoiding relates to particular situations. A child perceives that his speech in certain contexts is not as good as in others, or he thinks that specific situations require more from him than he is able to cope with – queuing in McDonalds, answering the register, talking on the telephone, for instance. So he avoids placing himself in those situations. He does not go out with his friends because he knows he will at some point have to stand in a queue and ask a stranger for a Big Mac and b's are hard to say. So he does not go. He is always late for school because he cannot say 'Miss' when the teacher calls his name on the register. He has few friends because he cannot make arrangements to meet them out of school, talking on the phone is just too threatening. So the hidden aspects of stammering can mean that some parts of a child's or adolescent's life are limited and increasingly restricted.

How the child sees himself One of the biggest problems with stammering is the long-term effect it can have on the child's view of himself. As we have seen in some of the examples above, the hidden aspects of the stammer can mean that he is not 'true to himself'. He does not say the words he really means, he chooses different food in a restaurant because he cannot say what he would like to eat, and so it goes on, day in and day out, until eventually his 'true self' is lost or hidden by the 'stammering self' and he comes to see himself as a stammerer.

Feelings We have known children who have developed several negative feelings associated with talking. Some are fearful of speaking in certain situations, will not answer in class, rarely argue or disagree with their peers because it puts too much pressure on their speech and they fear the consequences. Other children are very angry that they appear to have been singled out for this problem – the 'why me?' syndrome. They may be unable to articulate this anger but it can surface in other ways, for example, in their relationships with brothers or sisters, in their behaviour at school or in their play.

Stress Some children become quite stressed as a result of their speech and perhaps in their attempts to hide their difficulties. Once again the link between their speech and their feelings may not be obvious. As parents we are often made aware that all is not well with children of our own because they are acting differently from how we expect. They can be more aggressive or more withdrawn than normal. They may get upset for no apparent reason or seem generally out of sorts. Whatever the difference we know that something is wrong. The same observations apply to children with stammering speech. Their speech may be the source of anxiety which can result in a significant change in their normal behaviour.

Isolation Speech enables us as individuals to communicate with other individuals. If the speech breaks down or there is a fear associated with it, then that ability to communicate is impaired and an individual can feel isolated from those around him. A child who stammers may become isolated from his peers and this is sometimes reflected in the way he occupies himself in his leisure time. Instead of playing in a group, he chooses to spend time in his bedroom or he becomes interested in solitary tasks such as model making, reading, playing on the computer. We are not suggesting that these activities are in themselves bad, but when they are the only things in which the child is interested and he rarely engages in activities that involve interaction with others, then we would be concerned.

These lists are not meant to be a comprehensive account of all the types of stammering speech or hidden aspects of stammering that are possible, but hopefully they give the reader a flavour of the kinds of difficulties which are included under the single lable of stammering.

The varied nature of stammering speech is one of the inherent problems which beset those who work with and attempt to change it. There is no one type of stammering. It is rather like a pizza where you can determine the contents and the various toppings from a wide selection. Each one may have the same base but rarely are two the same and even if the toppings are similar it is almost certain that they taste different to those who have purchased them!

Normal or not?

In order to understand stammering in children it is necessary to think a little about how speech generally develops. Perhaps by focusing on the processes that most children go through we may have a better grasp of what goes wrong, or indeed if anything does go wrong, in a child who experiences stammering speech.

The gradual emergence of language is viewed by many as one of the joys of parenthood perhaps because it is one of the first more obvious signs of the developing inner world of the child. An infant will progress from the 'coos' and 'oos' of the early months to an enjoyment of strings of sounds produced in response to a carer or sometimes said just for the fun of hearing them. Usually within the first year a clear word is spoken and then, like a snowball down a hill side, language is acquired at an amazing speed. A toddler will soak up new words, trying them in a variety of contexts to check that he has grasped their full meaning and to test how they sound. Different types of words are learnt; nouns, adjectives, verbs and so on. The child then has the tools necessary to put words together in a meaningful way, as opposed to listing items. For example, 'Daddy, biscuit' becomes 'Daddy me want biscuit'.

Some children develop language in a slow methodical way, whereas other children accelerate through any or all of the stages. In some cases the onset of the process is late and then the child has some catching up to do. Other children may have difficulties with one or more particular aspects of language – a child can have problems remembering words, difficulties putting them in the correct sequence, or may not conceptualize that words carry meanings at all. These are difficulties that the child frequently sorts out with time but can often benefit from professional help.

With regard to fluency, once the child reaches the stage of putting words together in sequences there is potentially a problem with the flow and timing of speech. In order to produce a sentence, even a short sentence such as we illustrated above, the child needs a number of quite demanding skills. He needs:

• to have an idea of what he wants to say in his head. (Sometimes very young children will talk in a non-meaningful way. They are aware that it is their turn to talk, but have not sorted out what to say before they begin. Consequently what comes out is a string of nonsense to the listener, but the child is quite happy playing with sounds and words in an arbitrary way during his turn. This can also happen in children who are not using words. They may just enjoy the sounds of language and have fun 'pretending' to talk like their parents or older siblings.)

- to have an awareness that certain ideas can be represented by sequences of sounds i.e. words. To know and remember, for example, that b-a-ll is the round toy with which you play catch or football.
- to be able to select from the dictionary held in his head the words which accurately reflect what he wishes to communicate. This process actually becomes more difficult as the child develops because he learns new words and so has a bigger dictionary from which he has to make a choice.
- to be able to place the words in the correct order to convey the meaning of his idea and in a way which follows the grammatical rules of the language he is speaking. For example, the instruction 'daddy push me' cannot be conveyed if the word order is changed to 'me push daddy'. Nor does it obey the language rules if the order is changed a third time 'push daddy me'.
- to be able to remember the order of the words while engaged in speaking the sentence.
- to be able to place the sounds which comprise each word in the right order. (We know as adults when this goes wrong the results can often be quite amusing. For example, ramster and habbit and crack creamers.)
- to be able to place lips, tongue, mouth in the right position and shape in order to make the individual sounds of the word. All this is needed and needed quickly. The child does not have an endless amount of time in which to co-ordinate all this and the window of opportunity for his talking turn is often quite small. His listener may be involved in other activities, other toys, other friends and not be prepared to wait for very long while he gets his speaking act together.

When you analyse all this it never ceases to amaze us how it all happens with such apparent ease for most children. However, it is important to remember that the child is in the process of acquiring all these skills. They do need practice to perfect their speech and they usually do not get it right all at once. There is a period of time when these skills do not work together and a child's speech may be hesitant, lacking in flow and not fluent. It is hardly surprising, given all there is to know and do, that this phase is regarded as normal. This lack of fluency can result from learning any one or any combination of the skills we have outlined above. For example, not knowing the accepted word to use in a certain context can mean the child takes longer to think of a word to use, or may reword the whole sentence to work in one he does know. A child may forget his original idea during the process of articulating the individual words, he may confuse the order of the words or the order of the sounds and need to take time to think the process through again. As adults we do not expect children to be able to perform new skills perfectly on the first, second or even third occasion. Neither should we expect children to master the fluency of speech immediately they begin to speak. Children usually experience a period of non-fluency as they acquire all the varied and complex skills involved in speech. We should be prepared for this stage and not make the giant leap towards assuming they are stammering.

A short history of stammering

Although we have no idea who was the first stammerer, there is evidence of stammering as far back as 2,500 years ago in an extract of Chinese poetry by Laotze. Many scholars believe Moses was a stammerer, although the original account in Hebrew suggests slow and sluggish speech. Certainly both the Bible and the Koran have accounts of Moses referring to his speech difficulty as an argument against his appointment as leader of the Jews. There is evidence of stammering in the 20th century BC as some hieroglyphics have been found indicating that the word 'nit-nit' referred to stammering. In classical Greece Demosthenes was said to have worn leaden plates on his chest and placed pebbles in his mouth to alleviate his speech problem. (Don't try that one at home, kids!) In addition we know that stammering occurred in Roman times. For example, a stammer features among the Roman Emperor Claudius's many difficulties. In fact the Romans seem to have been very familiar with stammering, and even had a family name for it, 'Balbus'. As we move through the centuries stammering continues to be documented. Avicenna, the Arab physician described the difficulty in some detail one thousand years ago and suggested some treatment techniques. Therapeutic advice was also given by Mercuralis in 1583 who believed fear to be a major precipitating factor and therefore recommended a calm, regulated life style.

From the 1700s onwards the development of science played a part in the accounts and alleviation of stammering symptoms. The first actual treatment for stammering was documented in Greek times when a thorough cauterizing of the tongue was the vogue. In theory science had an impact on thinking about the nature and causes of stammering, but in practical terms the tongue still featured as the primary focus of medical intervention. So-called professionals advised all kinds of monstrous assaults on the tongue, including application of embrocation, gargles, cutting wedges from the base, inserting hot needles and severing of nerves, all largely without anaesthetic. Application of various mechanical gadgets was also advocated. These appliances involved constricting the throat, the jaw, the breathing, and strapping the tongue. Other professionals advised a more indirect approach suggesting among other things changes in life style, more exercise and improved bowel movement. We are glad to report a more enlightened approach these days!

Modern day therapies originated in Britain through the work of Victorian 'elocutionists' such as James Thelwell. These first therapists seemed to rely heavily on physical punishment of their clients. It is interesting to notice that around this time the first book was published labelling stammerers as nervous. (No wonder they appeared nervous when the treatment was so ferocious!) Later influences from America were integrated into therapeutic ideas. We have seen left-handed stammerers forced to use their right hands, stammerers singing instead of talking, the use of metronomes to regulate talking, and devices to prevent stammerers hearing their own speech. None of these methods appears to have produced the looked-for cure and we continue to do the best we can for those individuals who stammer as adults. Fortunately, for children the picture is much more hopeful.

Myths and legends

In comparison to early times we seem to have moved light years away from the misconceptions held by society and many professionals. We still have a long way to go but there are encouraging signs that people are beginning to understand what it means to stammer and seem more able to discuss it openly, rather than hide it away like a skeleton in the cupboard.

There remain however, a number of popular myths about stammering which in some instances are throw-backs to early times.

All stammerers are nervous In our conversations with the public and members of other professions we are often aware of a stereotypical view of people who stammer. They seem to be perceived by some as fearful of situations, other people and life in general. They have no self-confidence or belief in themselves and very often are thought to have been born that way. However, studies carried out over a number of years involving a great many individuals paint a very different picture. Stammerers are no more nervous, fearful, anxious, lacking in self-confidence than anyone else. In fact they are as different or as similar to any person you might meet in the street. So you are no more and no less likely to meet a stammerer who lacks self-confidence than you are to meet a fluent speaker who lacks confidence.

Stammerers are less intelligent Similarly there is a belief that because a person lacks fluency of speech his thought or intellectual processes are deficient in some way. Once again research has shown that stammerers have no greater problems in this area than anyone else.

Stammering has a physical cause Some people think that stammering is related to a physical cause. Perhaps this may have originated in early times when round about AD 20 Galen proposed that the four qualities hot, cold, wet and dry were the components of the four elements earth, fire, water and air. It was thought then that disease was related in some way to an imbalance of these elements. We rarely meet people nowadays who discuss stammering in this precise way, but occasionally in some cultures stammering is attributed to a predominance of hot or cold weather, or hot or cold food and drink.

There are also those who link stammering to some physical cause in the child themselves; they believe it is a result of muscle problems with the tongue, lips, jaws or palate, or see a relationship between the length or size of the tongue as important. Perhaps the tongue is too big for the mouth, the jaw length is too small or maybe the frenulum (the piece of tissue that ties the tongue to the base of the mouth) is too short resulting in a 'tongue-tie'. Once again we can see a link with some of the early beliefs about the cause of stammering. Generally in our experience there is nothing wrong with a child's articulators or mouth proportions. Occasionally we may note a co-ordination difficulty or a problem positioning the tongue or lips for a particular sound. But this can occur in any child and is not likely to be the cause of a stammer. However, we would take care to discuss and/or assess these aspects of the child's speech as a matter of routine when they visited us, to eliminate them as possible contributing factors.

Stammering can be caught Some people believe that stammering is like a disease or illness that can be transmitted from person to person. Adults recount experiences of having friends who stammered or of sitting next to Bob whose speech was a real problem. Then they made the link between their own difficulties, the individual they knew and their knowledge about disease. In fact stammering cannot be caught in that way. As we will see in the next chapter there is some evidence to suggest it is genetically transmitted and thus runs in families, but it cannot be caught through contact with others who stammer. This has implications for families too. We have met parents or couples considering parenthood who are concerned that one or both of them could pass on their speech patterns to their children or prospective children. The only way they could do this is through their genes over which they have little or no control.

Stammering is a deliberate act From time to time we meet people who think stammering speech is something the child does on purpose. It is seen as attention-seeking behaviour or as a deliberate act to get out of doing certain activities, or speaking situations. Very occasionally it is perceived as 'naughtiness' – as if the child is speaking in this way purely to annoy or provoke. When viewed in this light then the reaction is often to instruct the child to stop speaking like this and return to a more 'normal' way of talking. Consequently, children are told to stop and slow down, start again, take a deep breath or think before they speak. Very occasionally they may be reprimanded and punished for the way they speak. In actual fact we have rarely, if ever, met a child who stammers on purpose. It is certainly not a pleasant experience and there are few, if any, rewards associated with it. Also, stammering is not something which is easily controlled. We wish it were, it would certainly make our job easier! Once established it is very difficult to change, let alone eradicate altogether. So the child will find it very difficult to comply with these generally well-meant instructions.

Stammering is caused by some traumatic event A final myth to consider again concerns the cause of stammering. Interestingly, the Amish people of America believe that babies who are tickled under the chin go on to stammer. However, what we are concerned with here are events of a more serious nature. In our discussions with parents and clients we have been struck by the number of cases where the onset of stammering has been sudden and also linked in people's minds to a major event in their lives. The types of events which have been mentioned to us include tonsillectomy operations, death in the family, encounters with wild animals (at the zoo) and minor accidents.

Perhaps these events are significant in people's lives but they do not necessarily have any special significance in relation to the child's stammer. It often happens that an important event is associated in an individual's mind with their first observation of the child's non-fluent speech. The pattern of speech may have been present for a while but only noticed at around the same time the important event took place. In this instance the event and the onset of stammering are intrinsically linked in the person's thoughts.

Another possible explanation is related to the model of stammering we shall explain in the next chapter. Put succinctly, the child may have been experiencing difficulties or major changes in his life prior to the significant event, but the event itself has precipitated more obvious speech problems. Thus, the event itself is not responsible but is more like the straw which broke the camel's back!

Causes

As we have seen in the preceding section, there is much speculation regarding the nature and causes of stammering. In the world of speech and language therapy there are more books and studies on this very topic than our library shelves can hold. Since the early scientific experiments on the tongues of stammerers there has been a plethora of research dedicated to finding its cause. An examination of this literature shows the variety of factors which have been blamed for causing stammering: handedness, brain-wave patterns, delays in processing what is heard, co-ordination of speech muscles, parents, cultural and social factors, physiological aspects, anxiety and other psychological factors – the list goes on and on. We are frequently asked what we believe to be the causes of stammering and our response, like others' in the profession, is 'We don't know – yet'. There is much we do know and our knowledge is growing year by year but we have no definitive answer at the present time. Our best guess, based on the current state of information, is that stammering is a problem with the nerves and muscles which direct and control the organs of speech. This problem results in some interference in the timing of movements needed for speech. It may be that in some cases there is an inherited component or some difficulty with processing from the brain, which means that these children are predisposed to stammering. However, most children will become fluent as they grow older and become more mature because they do not react adversely to these tiny disruptions of speech.

2
Making sense of stammering

In this chapter we would like to share with you some of the information we have about stammering and highlight some of the questions which remain unanswered. Our main aim in this next section, however, is to tell you about a way of looking at stammering which enables us to work with parents and others in order to help the children who have these types of difficulties.

What we know about stammering:
the story so far

Much of the early work on stammering in children was carried out by three people who contributed a great deal to what we know about the development of fluency and non-fluency. They were Wendel Johnson, Oliver Bloodstein and Charles Van Riper. Each one carried out a number of studies to try and find out what factors were involved in stammering and in particular to map out how a child might move from having 'normal' non-fluent speech to stammering. Although the research that each one carried out was different, in general they analysed the speech of individual children at different stages and different ages. Based on that information they then put forward ideas about the process of development which all children might go through. (This is referred to as a 'cross-sectional' approach.)

As individual researchers these people had their own particular areas of interest:

• Johnson was interested in the difference between the problems of fluency encountered in children who would go on to be normal speakers and the difficulties experienced by those children who would later be labelled stammerers. He came to believe that the child's responses and the views of those around him played an important part in this development. For example, if Bridget is bothered by what people think of her she is more likely to worry about how others perceive her 'normal' little lapses of fluency. Whereas Briony, who does not care what others think and will do her own thing no matter what, will have little or no anxiety over her little lapses.

• Bloodstein, meanwhile, believed that the only difference in the speech of children who developed stammering was in the degree of difficulty, i.e. they merely experienced more of the 'normal' non-fluencies. He went on to propose four possible ways in which stammering could develop. For example a child of four may develop a particular pattern different from another child in primary school or a teenager or even the pattern of an adult.

- Van Riper, on the other hand, proposed five 'tracks' or routes which a child might follow. He described these pathways in terms of the kind of speech problems the child has and also how the child is feeling. Unlike Bloodstein before him, Van Riper did not see these 'tracks' as discrete ways. Thus, a 'Van Riper' child begins on one track and can turn off onto another track at any particular time. He is not destined to pursue one road and one road only but can choose a new direction, which may include speaking and/or feeling differently.

Looking at the research on the development of stammering a number of important issues emerge.

The child's development

It is important to view the child as a whole and to see whether the individual aspects of his development are keeping pace with each other. For example, it would not be in Megan's interests to think about her ability to speak fluently if she did not have the maturity to cope with social situations and would much prefer just being by herself and not talking to anyone else. If we do not keep the total picture of the child in our minds then, as we shall see later in this chapter, we run the risk of setting up an imbalance in the child's overall development. Of particular concern is the development of speech and language. Studies have shown that this is vital to fluency and, as we have already mentioned, the ability to think of words, construct sentences and so on keeps the flow of speech going.

The child's own feelings about his speech

From the beginning researchers have identified the child's attitudes to speaking as one of the key issues. It may be that the child has a keen awareness of his abilities in this area from quite a young age. Some children can be quite accepting of their own lack of perfection, knowing that given time aspects of their performance will change. However, for others their abilities never seem quite good enough, they do not match up to their older sibling, to what they perceive grown ups to require from them, or even to their own high standards. Certainly we have met children in the course of our work who have found their little lapses in fluency totally unacceptable. One young child even resorted to saying 'doobie, doobie, doobie' rather than utter any non-fluencies. In such cases this uncompromising attitude to normal non-fluencies can create tensions within the child which serve to make the difficulties more severe.

The reaction of others to his speech

How other people respond to the child's non-fluencies is another key issue. If he believes his teacher, brother or sister or parent is embarrassed or impatient when he speaks, then he may come to feel that aspects of his speech are not acceptable to others and will try to change them in some way to get a better reaction. If, however, a child is given time to speak and there is a general acceptance of his speech it can foster a similar attitude in the child. He will learn to be patient with himself and be more accepting that this is a difficulty which will pass in time.

Pressures in the environment

As adults we are all aware we do not exist in a vacuum. All manner of things affect how people feel and act, including for some of us how we speak and think about the way we speak. We know that when we are tired or anxious our speech is affected (and we are speech therapists – what hope is there for the rest of the population?). So it is for children: situations in which they find themselves, people around them and demands which are made of them all contribute to their ability to control their behaviour, including speech.

The type of fluency problems experienced

Obviously the more dysfluency the child encounters, the more he will have to cope with. Some children will have an in-built mechanism for dealing with a lot of non-fluencies and will manage very well. However, other children do not have such resources and may find even small amounts of dysfluency difficult to cope with. Aside from the amount of stammering speech, the type of dysfluency can also be significant. For example, a momentary pause or hesitation which appears as a silence will be less disruptive than a dysfluency in which the child prolongs a sound for several seconds or repeats a number of words over and over again.

A look at the literature

A number of interesting areas have been the subject of debate in the research over the years. They fall under two main headings – nature and nurture.

Genetics

Is stammering actually a problem that runs in families? Can we put the occurrence of stammering down to 'something in the genes'? A number of studies have been carried out on the genetics of stammering. A summary of what we know in this area suggests there is a significant factor related to heredity. Let us look at the findings.

- Stammering is three times more common in families where stammering already exists, when compared to other families with no history of dysfluency.
- Stammering is more common in relatives of people who stammer than in the population as a whole. In general, the incidence of stammering is about 1 per cent, but this rises to a staggering 14 per cent among relatives of those who stammer.
- There does not appear to be a connection between severity and the number of people who stammer in a family (i.e. if a mother has a very severe stammer the number of her offspring who stammer would be no greater than if she had a mild problem).
- If there is a female in the family with a stammer then there is a greater occurrence of stammering in her relatives than in relatives of a male stammerer. Thus, if your gran on your mother's side stammered it is more likely that the relatives on that side of the family will inherit the problem. If, however, granddad had stammered or gran on your father's side, then the likelihood of relatives stammering on that side of the family is less.
- On a more positive note for the females, research shows that they have a greater chance of recovery than their male counterparts.

So on this basis we can say that there does seem to be evidence to suggest stammering is, in part, an inherited problem, with the sex of the individual also having an influence.

Parents and children

However, this is not the whole picture. We know that there are families where stammering does not occur despite the fact that dad, gran or uncle Terry had a very noticeable stammer. We also know that there are children who stammer but have no stammering relatives. Obviously something else is going on and researchers have investigated the environment of these children to try and identify a common pattern or possible causes. The results, to say the least, have been mixed! Let us look, for example, at what has been discovered about the way parents and children talk to each other.

- There are some studies which show that parents who have children who stammer are less tolerant of the breaks in their children's fluency than parents of non-stammering children.
- There are some studies which show that parents of children who stammer make more negative comments than parents of children who do not stammer.

On the other hand:

- There is evidence that both mothers of those who stammer and mothers of those who do not interrupt their children when they are not speaking fluently.
- There is evidence that there is little or no difference when you compare the parents of children who stammer with the parents whose children do not!

What are we to think?

What we would like to know about stammering

As you can see from the previous section there are a lot of contradictions in the research that has been carried out so far into stammering. The information we have shows us that stammering is a very complicated problem, with a number of varied factors appearing to affect whether or not it develops in children. It is certainly not the kind of problem that is going to have a straightforward answer. There is no little pink pill that we can give children to make it go away or one that we give to parents to prevent it happening at all. Indeed there are often times when we wish for a magic wand to produce such a result.

Children and their parents arrive at our clinics with lots of questions, wanting help for their particular areas of concern. Because of the state of the research into stammering, there are frequently questions to which we do not have answers. We can list the questions to which we would like researchers to find the answers:

If there is something in the genes of certain families, which gene is it? Given the state of scientific advances into work with genes perhaps, once the gene responsible for stammering is identified, then some preventive work might begin.

How strong does the genetic factor have to be? We know that heredity plays some part in stammering but as yet we do not know why and how it works. We need to know why the gene operates to develop stammering in some families and not in others. What does it have to combine with to create a potent mixture for the child?

How strong does the environmental factor have to be? Similarly, we can recognize that some aspects in a child's situation play a part in the development of stammering but we do not know how bad it has to get or what it has to mix with to create the 'bad medicine'. We know of some children who have been to hell and back in the space of their short lives but have no stammer. Other children appear to respond to a minor upset with non-fluent speech. So, what makes the difference?

How does stammering develop in children? As we have seen, the early work on developmental pathways took a cross-sectional approach, looking at different children at different ages and stages and, on the basis of that information, making general statements about the developmental pattern all children follow. We believe there are some problems with this method and would like to see researchers trying a 'longitudinal' approach. That would involve following a number of children as they grow up over several years and plotting the way in which their speech and fluency develops. Very little information has been collected in this way on stammering and we think it would be invaluable.

What are the key elements in recovery? We would like to be able to identify what it is that helps children resist turning those normal lapses of fluency into stammering speech. We know some of the factors that help (and we will be discussing them in more detail later) but we would like the complete picture. We would also like to know what elements are at work when children recover spontaneously. One minute they are very dysfluent and the next minute it seems the speech has sorted itself out – but why and how?

'Weighing up' the child who stammers

One way of looking at stammering in children has been proposed by an American speech therapist called Woody Starkweather. He was concerned about the amount of contradictory evidence on stammering and its development and attempted to unravel some strands of the tangled web of information to make sense of it all. What came out of this has proved to be a very useful model or tool which we can use as a starting point with any individual child.

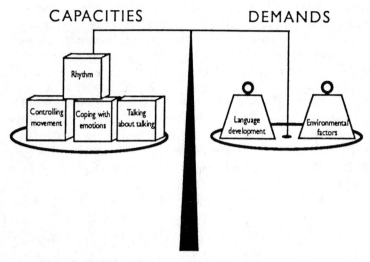

Figure 1: Weighing up the child who stammers

Starkweather begins with what we know about speech production and speech and language development in the young. He paints a picture of each child's ability to be fluent in terms of a balance or an old-fashioned pair of scales. Refer to Figure 1. On the left-hand side of the scales is a container into which we will place building blocks. These blocks will represent the child's speech and language and other aspects of his development. The number that a child has in his container will largely depend upon the stage of his development. Desmond, for example, is two and a half and has only a few building blocks on his scales. He has few words, struggles to put them together to form proper sentences and is not able to take turns as his parents do when they have a conversation or a discussion. As he gets older more building blocks are added to the left-hand side of the scales. Desmond learns more and more words, can vary what he says depending who he is talking to, can manage speaking to others, may take the lead and direct a topic of conversation. By the time he reaches the end of primary school education there are almost as many bricks in his left-hand dish as you would find on his mum's or dad's scale.

What about the other side of the scale? Well, Starkweather believes that the left side is counterbalanced by a set of weighted demands with which a child has to cope. These demands can be carried to the scales by people around the child, by situations in which the child finds himself and by the child himself. In Desmond's case (remember in the beginning he is only two and a half). Gran brings him a weight when she comes to see him. She asks him lots of questions about what he has been doing or what he has played with during the day or what he likes to eat for tea. This is difficult for Desmond to cope with, firstly because the questions seem to come at him all at once and, secondly, because he has difficulty remembering the answer (he cannot remember what he did three hours ago or the names of all the foods he likes to eat). Finally he sees Gran at the end of a long day and really just wants her to read him a story and not talk all the time.

The other big weight on Desmond's scales is that he is actually quite good at talking for his age. Even though he is only a toddler, he does put lots of words together and likes to show off with his talking sometimes. However, he likes to get it right and when those little lapses in flow and timing come along he can become a bit cross with himself.

Whereas we can almost guarantee that the left-hand side of the scales will become heavier with time (the older the child the greater the number of blocks), the right-hand side of the scales is not so predictable. Weights can be added as the child gets older: we will ask more of Desmond when he is eight than we do now at two. For example, his parents and Gran will naturally speak more slowly to him as a toddler but will speed up their speech as he becomes older. Also we are more accepting of some ways of talking. If Desmond asks for a 'dwink' his parents know what he wants and generally will comply without commenting on his mispronunciation. However, if he made the same mistake at nine or ten years of age his parents may have some comment to make! Another source of weight comes from events or situations in the child's life. The arrival of a new baby or starting school for the first time are events which most children will have to cope with at some point. The effort involved in coping, re-adjusting and maybe finding his place again, can mean that a child's energies are temporarily diverted, perhaps diverted away from coping with those little lapses in fluency. So when Desmond starts nursery, playgroup or school we should expect that any difficulties with fluency will become more apparent at that time.

Before we discuss what can be important issues on the scales for children, let us just be clear about what this model is telling us.

(1) Fluent talking should get better with age – providing the right-hand side of the scales remains constant, which of course it never does! Not only is it dependent upon keeping the right-hand weights to

a minimum, but also we cannot predict when and how a child will add building blocks to the left-hand side. Children seem in this, as in most things, to do it when they are ready and not before. It will not happen because other people think it should or because we deem it to be the 'right' time. The child's level of maturity and stage of development will largely determine when this will happen, despite our best efforts.
(2) The balance is not static. We should expect things, including speaking, to change. There will be changes in favour of the child's fluency, as he learns more language skills, and in favour of non-fluency when factors in the environment or inside the child put him under pressure.
(3) Maybe the best we can hope for is a child whose speech is frequently changing to meet new demands placed upon it. By that we mean we expect children to have times when their fluency is not as good as at other times and the model allows for that. We would be more concerned when a child is unable to adapt to the pressures being brought to bear on them; when he cannot add or move some of his building blocks to counterbalance the scales. As a result, the scales tip in favour of a more prolonged period of dysfluent speech.
(4) When the scales are tipped against fluency for a long time a child may struggle to right them. This struggle to lift the container on the left can result in 'struggling' speech. The lapses in flow and timing become filled with tension and pushing, in attempts to put them right. This is the pattern we know as stammering.

The building blocks

Let us now consider in more detail some of the parts that will make up the building blocks on the left-hand side of the child's fluency scales.

Rhythm

This is quite a tricky area and one where there is not a lot of information available. However, we do know that having a sense of rhythm helps us with language. Being able to spot a beat or a rhythmical pattern enables us to predict the timing of language and speech and we have already seen the link between timing and speech fluency. Rhythmical skills appear to develop in quite young infants. Babies, for example, will experiment with different strings of sounds and sequences with various beats when they babble. This is obviously an important phase for children to go through and should be encouraged. However, there are some babies who appear naturally quiet and do not engage in these noisy outbursts. Perhaps they are just quiet children, but we should be aware that there may be a need to provide them with some other form of experimentation or experience of rhythm when they are a little older. Musical tapes of various sorts are a useful resource: you can get children to sing, clap, stamp, making the beat more complex as they grow in confidence and ability. Home-made musical instruments can also be a source of fun when used to accompany pre-recorded music or to imitate different beats that mum or dad make.

Controlling movement

Talking involves using and co-ordinating lots and lots of very tiny muscles. The movements needed to make certain sounds are often miniscule – the difference between a 't' and a 'k' sound, for example, is a matter of a few millimetres. A child, therefore, needs to be able to plan in his head which sounds he needs to say a word and then send the appropriate messages via the nerve fibres to the muscles of his tongue, mouth, roof of the mouth and/or lips to tell them which ones are to move and in which order. As we have said before, this is such a complex process it is little wonder that things go wrong at times. Children who have the ability to control small sets of muscles are likely to be able to affect their speech muscles more easily. A speech and language therapist will be able to assess this aspect of a child's development and can suggest activities where there is a difficulty in fine muscle control and/or co-ordination.

Coping with emotion

As a child matures he usually becomes more able to cope in strange and unfamiliar situations. Thus, in terms of fluency, we can predict that young children will be more hesitant and unsure when faced with adults or children whom they have not encountered before. We have all met the little one who hides behind his parent or clings to his parent's leg when we attempt to talk to him. Meet him again in three or four years' time and we will rarely see the same reticence.

The ability to deal with excitement or extreme emotion generally also improves with age. Two-year-old Desmond will be so excited over his birthday party or trip to the zoo that his ability to do anything other than mundane, routine tasks is likely to be affected. This will apply to his speech too, of course. The excitement may outweigh his ability to think of words, to string them together, and he will probably experience more dysfluent speech. As adults we get close to this feeling when we have an issue pressing on our minds – we may be worried about someone or have just remembered an important task we should have done. The thought seems to fill our heads and we cannot concentrate on anything else until the problem is resolved. In these situations we can find ourselves withdrawing from conversation and conserving our energies and emotion for the difficulties in hand. Speech seems to require too much energy and concentration when other emotional issues demand our attention.

The final point to make under this heading relates to the emotion generated by the non-fluencies themselves. Perhaps we should have included this in the 'myths and legends' section as in some circles there appears to be an unwritten rule that stammering or dysfluent speech is too embarrassing to talk about. We have both met families in which the children's stammering speech was obvious to all concerned. In fact, the children were often struggling to keep the symptoms under some sort of control rather than letting them out. It is as if the children in these instances have perceived that what they were doing was so bad that no one could actually discuss it with them. Perhaps they noticed some subtle facial expression, or a change in body position or a look in someone's eye – whatever the reason, the issue and the emotion associated with stammering speech had been brushed under the carpet. Having said all that, there is a fine line to be drawn between creating a taboo about stammering and drawing children's attention to non-fluencies of which they have been blissfully unaware. We are *not* suggesting that children who do not react in any way to their little lapses should be made conscious of them. However, when children are reacting with struggle and push and/or shows by some action or expression that this speaking business is giving them a bit of bother, then we need to respond. Starkweather, the American speech and language therapist mentioned earlier, gave a lovely example of this in a talk we once heard him give. He said if a young child falls down on the pavement, grazes his knee and is in obvious distress, the parent or carer will go to the child and give him comfort, perhaps saying 'There, there' or some other words of reassurance. Similarly, when a child falls down in his talking, if the child is in distress we need to respond with the equivalent of 'There, there' and kiss his talking better! One suggestion we have used is to make a comment along the lines of 'My, that word was hard to say. Do you know I have words like that? Sometimes when I'm tired or a bit worried about something I forget my words or get stuck.' Or 'I especially have trouble with statistics.' Or 'I know your dad can never say thief.'

Talking about talking

Personally we have found that if we can talk about a problem to other people, then the problem seems less insurmountable than when we try and deal with it alone. That is not to say the problem disappears, it just helps to be able to discuss it openly with a sympathetic listener. The same principle appears to apply to children with non-fluent speech. If they are able to talk about the problems they are having with their speech then it helps them cope better. The problem does not necessarily go away, but speaking about it with someone may help children understand what is going on and reduce the anxiety which can arise. If children bottle up the feelings and worries they have, then this can create extra 'weight' that they have to carry about with them and does not help the overall balance of the scales. This was clearly illustrated to us by a young client we once met. At the age of two and a half he was experiencing a difficult period of dysfluent speech and appeared to be increasingly concerned about it. This was demonstrated as his usual outgoing nature became more and more indrawn; he began to prefer solitary play, his sleep patterns were disrupted and he talked less. Once opportunities were made to discuss what was happening in his speech and give him a better understanding then things improved considerably. His behaviour returned to normal and he began to make comments about his non-fluencies, for example, 'My words are a bit sticky today, Mummy'.

The weights

Let us now consider the right-hand container of our scales. You remember that this side of the balance consists of a set of demands which can originate from inside the child or be a product of his environment. We will think first of those demands which the child may generate.

Language development

As language develops it creates its own set of demands for the child. Consider William, 18 months old and only just beginning to talk. He knows between 30 to 40 words consistently, and so does not have many from which to make a choice. He speaks in very short phrases – in fact he has begun to put two words together to form little sentences. Obviously this does not demand a great deal of planning and words can 'double up'. For example, 'Me drink' can be a request for some milk or a statement to tell anyone who is interested what he is up to! William's speech sounds are also restricted. He cannot yet say some of the sounds we use in English: 'k' comes out as 't' and 'r' sounds like 'w', for example. Once again, his speech is simplified with some sounds 'doubling up' for others. For example, 't' is used for both 'k' and 's', so he says 'tight' for 'kite' and 'tee' for 'see'. Finally, he has not yet learnt the rules about when to speak, when to be silent, when to take a turn at talking, and how to make what you say match who you are speaking to. As a result he will talk while he plays and his little sentences seem to mirror all the actions of the toys with which he plays. He interrupts adults and will take his talking turn whenever he wants to say something. He also says inappropriate things in certain situations, for example, in the middle of a busy cafe he may point to a larger sized man and say 'Fatty man' much to the horror of his mum or dad!

Now look at William aged six. He knows hundreds of words by this time and so making a choice about which is the right one to use in a certain context is quite a difficult task. He speaks in long, complicated sentences and as a result has quite a lot of planning to do in his head to make sure the sentence comes out with the words in the right order, the letters in the correct sequence and spoken in the appropriate way. He is able to use almost all of the sounds of English (occasionally his 'r's are mispronounced in certain words like 'squirrel' or 'string') but people expect him to make his sounds in the right way. Sometimes when he does get his 'r's mixed up with his 'w's his gran corrects him or tells him to say the word again. Finally, he has some knowledge of the social use of language. He does not talk all the time he plays, but will choose the most important bits to share with others. For example, he will tell his parents or friends crucial aspects of his play, like 'I made a really scary monster from these pieces of Lego'. He knows he should not interrupt other people while they are talking and is beginning to understand what is appropriate to discuss with adults and what can be talked about with his friends.

Thus as William has got older his language system has become less and less restricted: his word choice is greater, his sentences are longer, his sound system has expanded. He has a greater knowledge and understanding about the rules of language and so there are greater pressures to make sure that his talking adheres to these rules. (This pressure, as we will see, can also come from adults around William, but at present we are only considering how William himself might add weights to his scales.)

So while the ability to use language can be a building block which appears on the left of our scales, we also see now that the ability to use language increasingly results in pressures of its own.

Environmental factors

In any child's life there are a great number of factors around him which potentially could add weight to his scales. We think that, in terms of significant people, parents and carers, friends or peers, and individuals at school are very important. When we look at specific environmental factors we would ask that you consider them in terms of those three groups of people.

Language (again!) The language used by the child, as we have already seen, is of great significance. The language used by those groups of people is also an important factor. There is evidence which shows that children try to use the same sort of speech as those around them (indeed, adults do this too!). So if William's parents speak quickly, he will try to talk at the same rate. This means he will not have enough time to think of his words, construct sentences or programme his speech muscles to do what he wants them to do.

He could have some problems taking his turn. Perhaps he plays with an articulate, domineering group of children who like to take the lead and direct William in their play. The children may speak quite quickly and their interactions take place in a quick-fire way, with lots of interruptions and talking over each other. For a child who is just learning to come to terms with the complexity of speech, this can be very daunting and a further weight on his scales.

In addition the language used by significant other people might be too complicated. Teachers may use vocabulary which William is unsure of or does not yet understand. The sentences are long and appear complicated and William cannot remember all the teacher has said or told him to do. Those scales get heavier by the minute!

The pace of life Apart from the speed of speech, the speed of life can also be a factor on this side of the balance. Perhaps William lives in a very busy household with constant toings and froings, comings and goings. It is William's perception that things are always done at great speed: he has to get ready quickly if the family are going out, he has to eat his dinner quickly so that the dishes can be cleared away, homework has to be completed in order to move on to the next activity. Phew! it all seems so tiring – and for William there is a sense of never being able to prepare for events or think about what is happening or what might happen. He is unable to prepare his thoughts, his actions or his speech.

Talk to me! There is one weight which comes from other people demanding speech from children. Adults and teachers do it a lot, children demand it of each other less. We talked about Desmond's gran and how she always asked him questions when she visited his house when all he really wanted was to be read to. That is the type of thing we mean. Situations in which adults will demand speech of children, instead of providing them with an option. The difference between 'What do you want for tea?' and 'I thought we could have sausages for tea today, but perhaps there is something you would like better than that?' In practical terms it is quite a small difference, but for a child who has had a long day, just wants to watch television and not talk, the difference can mean a lighter container and a more balanced scale.

Important events For young children even mundane everyday events can be exciting. However, as children grow older they become more discriminating and will only engage their emotional gears over certain things. We have been able to identify some key events which add weights to the scales: moving house, birth of a new brother or sister, changing schools, death in the family or of a close friend, losing a precious toy, marital discord and divorce. For any child these events are traumatic and may result in behaviour changes. For a child whose fluency is at risk we should expect these events to have a possible effect on fluency.

The effect of not being fluent It seems pretty obvious to say that stammering will have an effect on the child. However, non-fluent speech can evoke reactions in other people which the child might have difficulty understanding. Some people respond negatively: do not look at the child, look too much, appear uncomfortable, speak for them and so on. Others respond in a more subtle way, for example, giving the child more attention than normal, which still gives the child the message that the way he is speaking is different and unacceptable.

If the child is at the stage of being unaware that anything is wrong with his speech (and in fact he may be right and it is the adults who are wrong), then these messages will be very confusing.

'I like to get it right' We have mentioned the children who appear to set themselves very high standards. Sometimes these desires to get rid of the early behaviours of childhood originate from the children themselves. There are other examples which we have seen of children trying to behave like an older sibling and of course they cannot, being several years their junior.

For these children the process of growing up is particularly difficult because it is so unacceptable. They want to get it right from the beginning. The experience of normal non-fluent speech will similarly cause these individuals problems and adds a weight to their system.

Looking at the scales of a particular child

Points to remember:

(1) Each child is different. Worries for one child may not cause another child a second thought. As therapists we therefore approach each child with fresh eyes. We aim to create a picture of the individual's scales, the factors that are at work in that particular child. We do not attempt to make the set of factors outlined above fit the child. Some could be relevant while others are not and we need to find out which are which.

(2) The building blocks on the left-hand side of the scales will mount up as the child grows older. We may not be able to add bricks to that side of the balance or make the child acquire a new brick. However, there are ways in which we can help a child to make the best use of the bricks he has at any one time.

(3) The weights on the right-hand side of the balance often stem from the environment and, as such, are more easily shifted. While the blocks on the left are frequently difficult to change, we could try to lift some of the load created by the circumstances in which the child has to talk. That explains why we frequently work through a child's family and discuss strategies with school or nursery.

(4) Our ability to make change happen does not solely rest in our own hands. We know ourselves that as parents and carers we feel a great need to take responsibility for making things better and putting things right. However, despite the best will in the world, other situations, other people and other feelings in the child operate in their own right. We can only do our best, give it our best shot and hope.

(5) We need help. We have found that we get the best possible results when everyone concerned with the child cooperates and works together as a team.

3

The developmental stages of stammering (1):
Early dysfluency

In this chapter we will explore how stammering seems to develop and also look in some detail at how it may start. In the following chapter you will read more about the later stages of stammering. We expect you will find yourself identifying certain aspects of your own child's dysfluency as you read about each stage. Hopefully you will have a clearer idea as to whether his speech is actually a problem for him and if so, what sort of problem it is. As we will see later, dysfluency may seem very different through a child's eyes than through an adult's. However, even if you feel fairly sure that your child's speech is at a particular stage, we would urge you to continue to read about the other stages. This is because there are many issues which we discuss that are equally relevant at all stages but in order to avoid needless repetition we mention them only in relation to one.

In order to look at the development of stammering, it seems sensible to begin by looking at what we mean when we use the terms 'development' and 'developmental stage'. When we consider children, the word 'development' is generally thought to refer to an ongoing process, a movement from one state of affairs to another. Books on the subject will usually look at a number of key areas, such as physical, intellectual, language, social and emotional development, the development of personality and of morals.

When we talk about a developmental stage, what exactly are we thinking about? The term usually means more than just an increase in size and includes an increase in complexity. In other words it implies that something new and more involved is happening, rather than more of the same. If we consider physical development, for example, when a child is able to sit up alone, this involves a mastery of balance and a degree of independence which was not present when the child could only sit up with support. Another idea often associated with developmental stages is that they should happen at approximately the same age in most children and in a similar sequence. (Most children sit alone for short periods at around nine months of age and cannot sit alone before they can sit unsupported.)

So how does all this apply to the development of fluency and of stammering, opposite sides of the same coin? We have seen in Chapter 2 that the development of fluent speech in children depends on their ability to 'balance' their own capabilities (muscular, emotional, intellectual and rhythmical) with the demands placed on them by themselves, by others or by the situation they are in. As children get older they are generally more able to perform this balancing act and thus their fluency increases. Let us now consider whether there are identifiable developmental stages in children's fluency in the same way as there are, for example, in physical and language development. This presents us with some difficulty and perhaps helps to explain why it is often so hard to make sense of children's fluency or dysfluency. To begin with, fluency is never a new stage in a developing child: it is something which was there before. Rather then it is the *degree* of fluency which typically changes as children grow older – they get more of it! Putting an age to when these increases in fluency occur is also problematic. Taking the example of our own families, one child had a very high degree of fluency by the age of three, another was very dysfluent at times at the same age and beyond, yet neither was still dysfluent at five.

It would seem then that we cannot say children's fluency develops in a way which is predictable and systematic, and we cannot closely define common stages which most children follow at approximately the same age. Yet this chapter is called 'developmental stages of stammering' and therefore seems to imply an assumption on our part that those children who stammer are the same and that all stammering develops in the same way. Of course, we know that this is not the case. However, unless we tried to define some broad categories of development we would not be able to make any generalizations and writing this book would be an impossible task. In fact, we would have to write a different book for each dysfluent child! We therefore propose that whilst, in practice, clear-cut stages with obvious entry and exit points are rarely apparent, there are enough similarities to enable us to provide a broad overview of some of the things which happen at the different phases in the development of stammering.

Where does all this lead us? Well, we have chosen to look more closely at three phases of stammering which we are calling 'early dysfluency', 'borderline stammering' and 'confirmed stammering'. We say 'chosen' because, as we have already determined, in reality actual phases do not exist. Some specialists in the field discuss more phases than we do (Peters and Guitar, 1991, for example, outline five). The phases we will consider are those that we find helpful in our everyday work with children and young people. Unlike some other writers we do not feel able to assign specific age ranges to our phases for a number of reasons. First of all, it is too difficult! More importantly, it can also be misleading and confusing. As we have already discussed, whilst the majority of dysfluent children of a certain age may fit into one particular phase, a considerable number will not.

Early dysfluency

We have already established in an earlier chapter that we cannot give any answers (or certainly any which would hold up in a court of law!) to the question, 'why does my child stammer?' Another question we are often asked is '*how* and *when* does stammering begin?' Answering this gives us almost as much difficulty. Let us refer back to Chapter 2 in which we discussed the development of children's fluency. We established there that the speech of young children is certainly *not* fluent and that it is hard, indeed almost impossible, to differentiate between the dysfluent speech of children who will go on to be fluent and of those who will begin to stammer. Indeed the speech of individual children in both groups is often very similar. This is why we refer to this early stage as early dysfluency and not early stammering – we do not know enough to be sure we can split the two into their own separate compartments. We wish, however, that we did. Our job would be so much easier if we could have a list in which we check off ticks and crosses, rather like a quiz in a magazine. We could then come out with a score to tell us exactly at which stage the child is. Unfortunately, life's not like that!

Perhaps we should begin by looking at some examples of children who we would say are in an early stage of dysfluency. These are not descriptions of real people, but they could be. Instead we have tried to include some specific points, all of which we frequently see in our everyday work, in order to illustrate those points we want to make. You will notice that at this point we do not use the word 'stammering' or 'stuttering'. This is because we do not feel enough is known for us to be sure of whether this kind of speech is a phase of so called 'normal' development or whether it will become something more like 'real' stammering. Most of these children will not stammer when they are grown-up. In fact, Sheehan and Martyn (1966) tell us that up to 80 per cent of dysfluent children will become fluent without any help from professionals.

EARLY ETHAN
Ethan is just three years old. He is a lively little boy with lots to say for himself. He started to talk quite early. He now knows a lot of words and uses quite complicated sentences. Much of the time his speech

is very fluent. Ethan has never been a very good sleeper and although his sleep patterns are beginning to improve, he still doesn't like going to bed and will often wake up in the middle of the night. He wears nappies at night and quite often wets himself in the day time. He tends to be somewhat clumsy: his mum refers to him as 'an accident waiting to happen'. Just recently his speech has become quite dysfluent. This is more noticeable at certain times, especially when he is tired, excited or when he is trying to explain something complicated. He is the sort of child who wants to say *exactly* what he means, using the right words and explaining every single detail. Sometimes he gets quite frustrated when he is unable to express himself as he wants to, especially if he feels people are losing interest in his long and involved tale! He will stamp his feet and on one occasion was heard to say 'I can't say that word'. His dysfluent speech consists of repetitions of words ('Mummy, Mummy, Mummy, I've seen a bird in the garden'), of parts of words ('It was a bi-bi-big bird') and of sounds ('It made a n-n-n-n-n-n-noise at me'). Sometimes these repetitions seem to go on for ever! However, much of the time he speaks with a lot of fluency.

EARLY ELI

Eli is four years old. He was a little late in learning to talk and is only now using sentences. He still gets his words a bit muddled on occasions. He sleeps and eats well and has enjoyed going to the local nursery school since he started there two months ago, although the staff have commented that he is rather quiet. It was about the time of his starting there that his parents noticed his speech was not as fluent as it had been. Quite a few changes were going on for Eli at the time. His Dad started to work shifts and although he still saw quite a lot of his son, Eli never knew when his Dad would be at home and when he would be at work. His baby sister was just three months old and he wasn't finding it very easy to get used to not being the only child in the family. In fact his behaviour has been really bad lately. He can't be trusted to be left alone in the same room as his sister and he is having some awful tantrums (usually in the local supermarket!). Although the overall amount of the dysfluency is the same, just lately there have been times when Eli seems to be really struggling to get some of his words out, especially when Mum is busy with the baby or making tea. He doesn't seem to be particularly worried or even to notice his 'difficulties' although there have been one or two occasions when he's either not wanted to talk or won't finish what he is saying if he gets stuck mid-stream. His parents are understandably quite concerned, especially as other people are beginning to ask them what the matter is with Eli's speech.

EARLY EMILY

Emily is nearly four and a half. Her speech development has been average and she now speaks in sentences. She is due to start school in two weeks. Her three older brothers and sisters are there already. They have told her all about it and she's getting excited now. She's been for a visit and has got a new track suit with the school's emblem on it. She didn't go to nursery school but is used to leaving her Mum when she goes to the childminder's each morning. Emily's Dad used to stammer when he was younger, in fact he still does a bit, although usually it doesn't worry him. His stammer is worse when he's talking with a lot of people or to someone in authority, like his boss. At home it isn't seen as a problem, and is viewed as just the way Dad talks. Emily's brothers and sisters get on well with her most of the time, although like most children they all fall out from time to time. The household is quite busy with all the children. In the morning everyone has to be out by 8:15 and there always seems to be someone who isn't ready. Teatime is usually a pretty hectic affair too, everyone wants to have their say. Emily sometimes finds that when she talks people get impatient with her and interrupt her or tell her to 'spit it out' (especially her next brother up, who never shuts up!). Her Mum and Dad try to make sure she gets her two penn'orth in, but it isn't easy. Emily often repeats words or parts of words, or sometimes nearly the whole sentence. It seems to be a case of little and often with her, and she can be dysfluent anywhere and everywhere, even when she is really relaxed. The repetitions don't last long but there are a lot of them. She gives the impression that when she does get her turn, she's jolly well not going to give up! Her speech has been like this for about a year now. Everyone told her parents she would 'grow out of it' and they're still waiting for it to happen!

Ethan, Eli and Emily are all 'normal' children, different in some ways, similar in others. One thing that they have in common is that they all have dysfluent speech. None, any, or all of them may stammer as adults. We do not have a crystal ball and so we cannot say which of them will and which will not. We can, however, look at each child individually and identify some of the factors which may be significant for them. In Chapter 5 we will look at how parents and others can help to change the child's environment in a way which is more likely to help the development of more fluent speech. In this chapter we are concerned with understanding the factors themselves.

Obvious and hidden dysfluency

First of all we need to look more closely at what in technical jargon are known as the *overt* and *covert* aspects of dysfluency. The term overt really just signifies that something is out in the open, obvious or unconcealed, whilst the word covert implies it is hidden or disguised. If we are overt about a breakup of a relationship, for example, we are prepared to talk about it openly and honestly, rather than disguising the facts or pretending that nothing has happened. When we apply the term overt to dysfluency, we are talking about those things that can be seen and heard by others. The many and differing features of this kind of stammering (such as repetitions, struggle, poor breath control, extra movements of the body and so on) have already been described in Chapter 1. In its early stages, dysfluency is almost totally overt. What you see is what you get! In other words, the child may stumble, repeat or struggle over words but does so usually without awareness that he is doing anything out of the ordinary and therefore without making any attempt to disguise what is happening. He may occasionally become frustrated if his words don't come out exactly when he wants them to but usually this is very short lived and related only to a particular moment in time. Sometimes it is hard for us as adults to realize that a behaviour which *seems* to be so obvious does not concern the child and is often something of which he is completely unaware.

Perhaps we can explain this more easily if we look at our three examples. For the most part, dysfluency is not a problem to the children we have described. Ethan loves talking – his occasional frustration seems to be linked to not being able to tell his involved tale to an ever-listening audience. Eli, although showing an increase in his overt fluency, rarely seems aware of it. Emily just battles on whenever she gets the chance!

The overt part of early dysfluency can offer us a number of clues as to whether the child is more likely to proceed to the next developmental stage (borderline stammering) in the future. When we see a child in clinic we look for a number of factors in our assessment of his *overt* symptoms. As you read through our list, however, we urge you not to be ticking off boxes in your head – this is only one small part of any assessment a speech and language therapist would make. If your child seems to show many of the points we are illustrating, it does not necessarily mean that he will go on to stammer for the rest of his life. So please, proceed in your reading with caution!

Points to consider in the child's speech

Speech and language development

There have been many conflicting views among clinicians and researchers as to whether children whose language skills are later in developing are more at risk of developing a stammer than those who develop language at an early or average rate. Unfortunately, yet again, our own answer has to be 'we don't know'. However, if we think of the scales model, then we feel this is an important area for us to assess in any child we see. Children whose building blocks are high enough in other areas for them to cope with the demands (or weights) they receive or impose on themselves, may still retain a high level of fluency despite some difficulties in their speech and language. Another child whose building blocks in other areas are less well developed, may find that their poor language skills tip the fluency balance and they become dysfluent.

However, there is more to it than this. Sometimes children who have advanced expressive language skills (who, for example, have a large vocabulary and mature sentence construction at a younger than average age) are also more at risk of being dysfluent for a number of reasons. They may not be as highly developed in other areas. Perhaps they do not have the fine motor skills which they need to co-ordinate the muscles of breathing, make sound and form sounds into particular words. They know what to say, the words to use and the order in which to use them but physically find they cannot say what they want to at the same speed as they might wish. The end result may be some disruption in the timing of their speech production: in other words, dysfluency. The same outcome can be seen in such children for other reasons. For example, perhaps they have good language and co-ordination skills but do not feel, for whatever reason, that their contribution is important and so it may come out in a rather faltering way.

If we look at our examples of Ethan, Eli and Emily, what do we discover? Ethan has good language skills but perhaps puts pressure on himself to 'get it right' when he speaks. There seem to be signs that his physical skills are less well developed. Perhaps the dysfluency in his speech is connected to both his own desire for perfection in talking and the current mismatch in his language and his physical skills. As he gets older and more of a balance develops in these skills, maybe the dysfluency will lessen. Eli's language development appears to be a little slower – maybe this is a factor as he struggles to express his ideas, especially when he is also coping with a lot of conflicting feelings about himself and those around him. And what of Emily? Language development does not seem to be a particular issue with her, although she finds it harder when she has to try and say all she wants to in a limited amount of time, before one of her older brothers or sisters tries to take over!

Amount of dysfluent speech

As we have said previously, the speech of most young children is often far from fluent. However, the amount of dysfluency in a young child's speech may be one clue in deciding what sort of difficulty the child is experiencing. There are two areas we feel are important to pay attention to. The first is the overall level of dysfluency, of whatever kind. This would include the more common repetitions of words and phrases as well as repetitions of parts of words, hesitations, struggle to say a word and the stretching out of a sound for longer than average time. The second area of interest is the actual dysfluent moment. If the child, for example, repeats a sound such as the 'p' sound in 'pig', does he typically do it once or twice or does he often do it seven or eight times?

Back to our examples. Ethan has a high level of fluency most of the time but when he is dysfluent, the actual moment can be quite drawn out. Eli's overall dysfluency has remained the same; it is rather its nature which changes. With Emily, the overall level of dysfluency is quite high but the actual moment remains fairly short.

Type of dysfluency

We also want to know what the dysfluency is like. Certain types of dysfluency are more common in all children, whereas others are more likely to be typical of the early stages of stammering. Generally speaking, we are more concerned if there is a lot of tension associated with the dysfluency. If the child, for example, repeats sounds in a slow relaxed way we are less perturbed than we might be if the repetitions are very rapid and strained. The former seems to indicate that the child is perceiving the disruption in his speech as something to be concerned about and is struggling to do something about it.

In our examples, both Ethan and Emily tend to have fairly relaxed repetitions most of the time with just an occasional more tense dysfluent utterance. Eli, on the other hand, is beginning to show more signs of struggle and tension in his speech.

When the child is dysfluent

Most children's speech is more dysfluent when they are tired, ill, excited or upset. So if we hear that this is the case with an individual child we are seeing, we are not overly concerned. If, however, we find that the child's speech is worse when he is in a particular place or with a particular person, then we might be more worried. We feel that this could be an indication that the child is becoming more aware that something is wrong with his speech and is anticipating that some people or places may be more difficult for him. We will discuss this in more detail later.

In the children we have described we also notice differences in when their dysfluencies occur. Ethan is typical of most children, being more dysfluent when tired or excited, but he also has difficulties which seem to be related to his own desire to say things 'just right'. Eli is more dysfluent when he finds it harder to get attention – for instance, when his Mum is involved with something or someone else. In Emily's case, there seems to be no particular pattern that we can see.

How long the child's speech has been dysfluent

It may seem rather obvious when we say that we are more likely to be concerned about a child's dysfluency the longer it has been apparent – but we'll say it anyway! However, as with all the other factors we are discussing this is only one part of the jigsaw. While a child who has been dysfluent for a year is often of more concern than the one who has been dysfluent for only six months, we are also interested in the *pattern* of the dysfluency. Has the frequency and amount of dysfluency remained the same or got worse, or has there been a degree of variety, with good and bad days or weeks? Has the type of dysfluency changed, is there now more or less tension? Are the good periods getting longer or are the bad periods becoming more frequent?

What can we say about our examples in respect of the time the dysfluency has been apparent? Ethan's dysfluency is relatively new but he does have a lot of time when it is not present. Eli, too, hasn't been dysfluent for long and although the amount of dysfluency seems about the same, the nature of his difficulties does seem to be changing with the introduction of more tension into his speech. Emily has been talking in much the same way for about a year now, nothing much has changed, for better or worse.

As we attempt to look at the three examples in more detail, breaking down their overt dysfluencies into particular categories, we begin to see how complex an area dysfluency can be and how difficult it is to make sense of. And we are only just beginning! There are other things to consider. We are interested in far more than what we observe in a child's speech. It is important that we try to understand the child himself and see if we can make sense of the dysfluency with reference to the individual. What kind of things might be important for us to think about in this respect? In the points we make below, we will refer to children we have had contact with in our own work, rather than return to our fictitious Ethan, Eli and Emily.

Points to consider in the child himself

How the child feels about speaking

It is interesting not only to know how the child feels about his dysfluency but also how he feels about speaking in general. Is it something he enjoys, does a lot of, feels easy about? Is he a chatty or a quiet child? Does he engage others mainly through speech or does he prefer to be more active in relationships and to 'do' rather than 'say'. Does he have times when he would rather not talk but would prefer just to 'be'? Unless we try to get some sense of the child's feelings about talking it is hard for us to tell if anything has changed if he becomes more dysfluent. Take Simon, for example, who was always a fairly quiet child. He wanted to say things when he wanted to and not when others demanded speech from him. His mother, however, was a more extrovert, chatty sort of person who liked to hear her son talking. She had no other children and when Simon came home from nursery she understandably longed to know what he had been doing, who he had played with, whether he had eaten his dinner, played in the sand and so on. Simon on the other hand just wanted some peace and quiet, a chance to play with his toys, watch television or look at a book. His mother worried that the dysfluency was the cause of Simon's quietness but on reflection she came to see that this was just the sort of child he was. In fact, in this respect he was very similar to his Dad, a more reflective, self-contained sort of person.

How the child feels about the dysfluency

As we have already discussed, one of the characteristics of the early stage of dysfluency is that the child is usually unaware of any difficulty in speaking and if he does have some knowledge of it, it is usually only fleeting and does not concern him unduly. The child may perhaps feel some frustration when he is unable to say things quite as easily as he might wish, in much the same way as all of us become frustrated when we cannot recall a word which is on the 'tip of our tongue' or cannot put a name to a face that we know well. This frustration may be expressed in a variety of ways. Mark, for example, would shrug his shoulders, take a deep breath and then start again. Susie would merely 'tut', as if acknowledging that she was having a bit of trouble. David sometimes banged his fist on his leg. Saleem would occasionally say 'I can't say it'. There are two things which differentiate this stage from the next phase of dysfluency (borderline stammering). The first is that the child's frustration is associated with the actual moment of the dysfluency. He does not anticipate that a word is going to be difficult to say; there is no flashing light in his brain which signals 'Oh no, trouble ahead, action needed!' Secondly, the feeling he experiences does not continue after he has said his piece. When the word is finally said, the frustration begins to go and rarely lasts for much longer.

What is going on in the rest of the child's life

Speech is not something that happens in a vacuum, separate from the rest of our lives. How often people say things like 'What's up? You sound really down', or 'You're sounding cheerful, have you won the lottery?' How we feel is often reflected in how we speak. So too, the things that happen around the young child can affect his developing fluency. Change, in particular, can be very difficult for some children to deal with. Some will sail through major upsets in their lives with no obvious difficulties of any kind. Others react strongly to even a minor alteration in routine.

So what sort of changes are we talking about? There are the changes that most children will have to experience in their early lives, such as going to a childminder, to nursery or school, the birth of a new baby. There are others that only some will experience, such as moving house, a change in life style due to unemployment, arguments at home, a period in hospital for parent or child, the separation or divorce of parents, the death of a loved one and physical or sexual abuse. Other changes may be less obvious but cause the child unhappiness or stress: for example, an older brother or sister leaving home, a friend moving away from the area, the loss of a favourite toy. Changes do not have to be negative. Many parents notice that their children have physical reactions of one type or another at times of high excitement. We remember how one of our children, who suffered from asthma, would always be ill at her own or others' birthday parties. The parents of one of our clients were very grateful that we had pointed out that their daughter's speech (which had improved a great deal over the previous few months) might get worse for a while as Christmas approached. It did (in fact she became *very* dysfluent) but the parents felt that the distress they experienced at this occurrence would have been much worse had they not been prepared.

Yet other changes which affect the child may be those of which adults are not even aware. Sometimes the child's reaction to the change is immediate and obvious, at other times it is delayed or hidden.

As in adulthood, children cope with change in their own particular ways. Some regress to an earlier stage of development and may for example begin to wet the bed after some time of being dry at night. They may become faddy about eating or develop fears of the dark, animals, going to bed and so on. Others change their behaviour. They become more introverted and clingy in an attempt to hang on to some sense of security. Some act out their upset and confusion and start to behave uncharacteristically. Others become dysfluent. Kirsty's dysfluency started after the death of her father. As she gradually came to terms with her grief, so the dysfluency lessened. Beth's difficulties seemed to start when her mother started work and she was left with a childminder, despite the fact that she always enjoyed going there. Everton's jealousy at his sister's birth seemed to be one of the factors in the onset of his dysfluency.

What home life is like

There are stresses and strains in the lives of all families. In today's world, family life seems to be getting busier, certainly if our own families are anything to go by. There are the demands that work brings, the need to work hard, often for long hours, times when it may be necessary to work away, to bring work home, either physically or emotionally, to be seen to be doing a 'good job'. Then the daily chores have to be fitted in, the tea made, the washing done and put away, the floors cleaned. On top of this we often try to be 'super parents', taking our children to after school activities, having their friends to tea, practising their reading with them, helping them learn new skills or do their homework, encouraging them to do something other than sit in front of a screen of one type or another. Sometimes, in our own families, we have the feeling that we are always busy: we lead our lives in a continual rush from one thing to the next. Often there seems to be no time to take stock or to spend time just 'being' with one another. These, and other factors about home life, will be discussed more in Chapter 5 when we look at how parents can best help their dysfluent children.

Summary

In this chapter, we have mentioned three stages of stammering development: early dysfluency, borderline stammering and confirmed stammering. We have given a comprehensive overview of early dysfluency and of the factors which may be apparent at this stage. In the next chapter we will go on to discuss the other two stages in similar detail.

4

The developmental stages of stammering (2):
Borderline and confirmed stammering

In this chapter we will explore how stammering can develop from a mild disruption in the timing of speech which does not give the child undue concern, into the more problematic stages of borderline and confirmed stammering.

Borderline dysfluency

What do we mean by 'borderline stammering'?

The word 'borderline' is used in everyday speech to indicate a transition from one thing to another. This idea fits well with our own feelings of this stage in the development of stammering. It is now that we need to be more aware of the *hidden* (or *covert*) part of stammering. The child is, at this stage, no longer unaware or unconcerned about his speech. It is likely to begin to be seen by him as a problem, to some extent and on a few occasions at least. The child may develop negative emotional reactions (for example, embarrassment or annoyance) connected with speech, and perhaps starts to anticipate difficulties in speaking. This developing awareness can also bring with it an attempt to hide or avoid the stammering behaviours.

Having established in principle what we mean when we talk of borderline stammering, we will now outline some typical case examples to help illustrate some of the points which will then be discussed in more detail.

BORDERLINE BRIAN

Brian is eight years old. His speech has been dysfluent since he was four. Until very recently it has not been a problem for him. His parents have been no more than a little concerned as the dysfluency has been mild and generally seemed to occur when Brian was upset, excited or particularly involved in what he was saying. He has always had a lot to say and until recently his dysfluency never stopped him saying it. The GP had said the dysfluency would slowly disappear as Brian got older and his parents felt reassured that this would be the case. However, in the last few months a couple of things have happened which have upset them. Brian came out of school one day looking down in the dumps. It wasn't until bedtime, however, that his parents managed to find out what was the matter. Some older children had been talking to Brian at playtime and had started to laugh at him, asking why he talked like that. Brian didn't understand what they meant and didn't know how to respond. Since then, Brian, who had always loved school, had on occasions said that he didn't want to go, or he had tummy ache. He did not relate his anxieties to the teasing incident but his parents felt they might be connected, especially as their usually talkative child was also becoming quieter at home.

BORDERLINE BETH

Beth is ten. Her speech has been dysfluent for as long as her mother can remember. Her parents separated reasonably amicably when she was two and she sees her Dad on a regular basis. Her mother remarried a couple of years ago and Beth has a good relationship with her stepfather. The dysfluency has never really bothered Beth and although she has been aware of it for some time it has been a bit of a nuisance rather than a problem. She is a popular girl and seems to get on well with most people. Her parents have noticed that she is stammering on more words and that some sounds seem to be more difficult to say than others. Beth has on occasions changed a word to one she found easier to say (for example, instead of saying she was ten, she said she would be 'eleven next birthday'). She seems to say 'um' and 'er' more often than most people too, as if she's not always sure of what she is saying. She admits to being more concerned about her speech and has asked her mum if she can get help.

BORDERLINE BASHIR

Bashir is six. He has always been a fairly quiet child, happy to play by himself. His dysfluency started about a year ago, shortly after he returned from a trip to Pakistan with his Dad and his older brother. To begin with, he would frequently repeat sounds at the beginning of a word and sometimes stretch out the middle of a word. Now he seems to stammer less overall but sometimes he gets really stuck – on occasions he looks very tense and it may take him several seconds to say a word. Starting off a sentence can be particularly hard. At times you can even see the veins stand up on his neck when he talks. Occasionally he has started to close his eyes or bang his fist on the table when he is finding a word hard to say. At other times, he does not seem able to express himself as well as he used to – it's as if he's not saying exactly what he wants to. When he is struggling over a word, he might attempt to stop what he is saying. His family always try to persuade him to finish and wait patiently for him to say what he wants to. However, they are beginning to worry that other people may not be as understanding.

Icebergs

Before we go on to discuss some of the features of this stage of stammering, we feel that our understanding of the development of the hidden part of stammering will be helped by comparing stammering to an iceberg. Sheehan, a famous American speech therapist, first described it in this way. We all know that the distinctive feature of an iceberg is that part which is above the water and visible, whilst the rest is below the water, not immediately obvious and therefore of more concern. If we consider the 'stammering iceberg' of a child who is in the early stage of dysfluency, it is almost totally above the surface. Little or nothing is hidden or covered up. In the borderline stammering phase, the picture begins to change. The part below the surface begins to grow as the child starts to be aware that his speech is different and attempts to do something about it. (See Figure 2.)

Features of borderline stammering

As we have stated, the key to borderline stammering is the change in the child's awareness and concern about his speech. As he begins to feel something is wrong, he tries to do something about it. How might we recognize that this is happening? We will now look at a number of areas in which this change may be seen. Not all of the factors we describe will, of course, be seen in all children.

The child's overt stammering The actual stammering behaviours may change at this time in a number of ways:

- The *nature* of the dysfluency could change. The child may start to 'struggle' when he speaks. He feels that the words do not come out easily so he starts to try to push them out. Whereas previously his dysfluency sounded fairly relaxed, there is now more associated tension. The child may 'push through' the sounds, making them harsh and strained. In our examples, this was the case with Brian, the tension being particularly visible in his neck.

- The *amount* of the dysfluency could change. It may become greater as

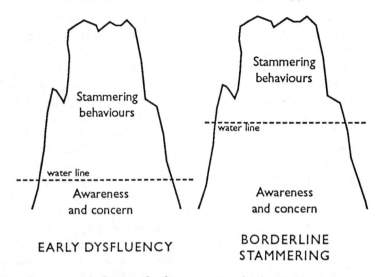

Figure 2: Stammering Icebergs

the child begins to anticipate having difficulty and so puts more effort (tension) into what he is saying. This is the case with Beth. It may, on the other hand become less, as the child starts to try to hide the stammer. It is like this with Bashir. Although his stammer has become more tense, it also happens less frequently. However, there are signs that he is not using the words he really wants to. Consequently his thoughts are not being expressed as completely as he is capable of. Another way in which the *amount* of dysfluency may change is that the periods when the child is fluent start to occur less often than before, while the times he is dysfluent happen more frequently.

- *When and where* the dysfluency occurs could change. This can happen as the child *anticipates* difficulty. As we mentioned in Chapter 3, the child who is at the stage of early dysfluency does not expect to have any problems saying the things he wants to. The borderline stammerer, however, may anticipate that there are problems ahead. This anticipation is sometimes linked with a particular word and the child perhaps starts to perceive that certain words cause him more difficulty than others (because the word is long or short or starts with a particular sound etc.). Sometimes the word on

49

which difficulty is anticipated is changed (Beth, for example, felt that ten was hard to say and changed it to 'nearly eleven'). Anticipation can be linked to a specific person (the teacher, the child who teases him, the brother who doesn't let him get a word in edgeways). A particular place can be the focus for the anticipation (his friend's house, grandma's house, school). In our examples, Brian seems to have been anticipating problems in talking at school. It may be a particular activity (cubs, football lessons) or a situation (talking with adults, or older children) with which difficulty in speaking becomes linked.

In some children we see a change in the level of dysfluency over the school year. A child we knew called Diane showed a fairly common pattern in her speech. It tended to be better during the school holidays, got worse at the start of a new term but improved within a few weeks. After that it would begin to worsen as the holidays approached when it would again improve. We might speculate about why this happened (but remember that it is just speculation). It could be that Diane coped better in the holidays, when she was faced with fewer demands. As she got into her stride again her speech improved but then worsened as tiredness began to effect her. If we refer back to the 'scales' image, outlined in Chapter 2, we have here an example of demands (or weights) outweighing Diane's building blocks at certain times.

- *Accompanying movements* could appear. Sometimes the struggle which occurs as the child tries to push the sound out involves other parts of the body too. You may remember that Bashir banged his fist. Other children we have known have done things such as screw up or blink their eyes, fidget excessively or tap their feet.

- *Extra words or sounds* could be added. Some children find that by adding extra words or sounds into their speech, they are able to say the feared word more easily. In the case example, Beth used 'er' and 'um' more than average. Other children use words or short phrases either in the middle of what they are saying (for example, 'I went to the, you know, circus') or as a starter, or run in to the beginning of a sentence (for example, 'actually I've just finished my homework').

Extra movements, sounds or words may develop almost as a 'magic trick'. If you think back to your own childhood, you perhaps remember using similar devices yourself. One of us remembers walking back from school and both estimating and then counting the number of strides it took to get from one road junction to another. If the estimate and the actual count were close in number, she would tell herself that whatever problem she had would be resolved (for example, that she had passed the maths test or that her friend would be understanding of some misdemeanour). It could be that some of these extra behaviours develop in the young dysfluent child in a similar way: the child finds, for example, that on one occasion, screwing up his eyes seems to help him to say a word more easily, so that the next time he anticipates difficulty he employs the same technique.

The child's behaviour

There could be a number of changes in the child's behaviour which can alert us to the fact that he is becoming more aware and concerned about his speech:

- the child may become less outgoing, withdraws more into himself or talks less (as in the case of Brian);
- the child's behaviour may change in other ways. For example, he becomes moody, aggressive, argumentative, more sensitive to frustration or criticism, cries more easily than before, and so on;
- the child may avoid doing things involving talking which he has previously been happy to do. This could include such things as doing errands, talking to visitors, asking or answering questions in class, volunteering to read out or to take part in an assembly.

The child's reaction to the dysfluency

A number of factors are contained under this heading:

- Immediate and/or open reactions. The child may be able to talk about difficulties in speaking (see Chapter 2 for more discussion about this). Colin told his Dad he couldn't say some words properly. The child may ask questions about his speech. In the cases we have outlined in more detail, Brian wanted to know why people laughed at how he talked, whilst Beth asked if she could have some help with her talking.
- Hiding the stammer. Sometimes children may begin to sense that something is not quite right about how they talk and try to hide it. Bashir, like Beth, seemed on some occasions to be changing the words he used. At other times Bashir wanted to just stop what he was saying altogether. Another child, Jaspal, put on funny voices or strange accents in an attempt to disguise the stammer. Jason missed out sounds with which anticipated having difficulty, making his speech sound quite strange to his listener but in his own mind reducing the struggle he was having to say words. William's ploy was sometimes to pretend to forget what he was going to say or to say he

didn't know the answer. Some children try to hide the stammer by non-verbal means; they may shrug their shoulders, make gestures, mutter meaningless sounds and so on, rather than speak. They may even, on occasions, ask someone to talk for them.

The child's feelings about the dysfluency

When we discussed early dysfluency, we talked about how any negative feelings that the child might experience at this stage were linked to the moment of stammering and rarely lasted more than a few seconds. In borderline dysfluency this can start to change. The feelings may become more intense and can last longer. The sort of negative feelings vary from child to child and individual children will respond differently at different times. The reaction is not necessarily linked to the overt severity of the stammering. An episode of stammering which appears mild to an observer may upset a child on one occasion when a more overtly mild episode upsets the same child much more on another day.

What do we mean when we talk of negative feelings? These can be many and varied and include concern, embarrassment, anger, frustration, anxiety, fear, loss of control, to name but a few! However, as we will see in the next chapter, it is important that as adults we try to separate our own emotions about the child's dysfluency from our assumptions about what the child might actually be feeling. We may, for example, *assume* that a child feels embarrassed or frustrated when he stammers in the shop asking for an ice cream, whereas in fact the emotion that the child is actually experiencing is annoyance that the shopkeeper has sold out of the particular flavour he wanted.

Sometimes the child's negative emotions are 'diverted' and, rather than experience them directly, they are experienced physically. One of our children, for example, hated his clarinet lessons at school. He had been keen to learn to play, an instrument had been loaned him, money was spent on music. He got praise from his family when he seemed to have quite an aptitude for playing. He gave a few hints that he didn't enjoy playing and needed to be nagged into practice. This, however, was fairly typical when he was asked to do anything which required effort! It wasn't until he started to feel ill every Thursday morning but always recovered for Friday (when he had games) that we began to realize what was happening. The illness disappeared when, after discussion about his feelings towards playing, the clarinet was returned to school. In the same way, emotions about stammering may be realized in uncharacteristic behaviour, as we have already discussed, or in physical symptoms. These are not deliberate, but rather the child's way of trying to cope with something he finds difficult. In the example of Brian, his tummy ache was a symptom of his feelings about the teasing he had experienced at school.

Additional points about borderline dysfluency

(1) Many of the things which we have described occur with as much frequency and for a variety of reasons in children who do not experience any problems with fluency; they are part and parcel of growing up. This makes our task all the more difficult since how do we know when a particular behaviour is connected with fluency and when it is not? While there are no easy answers, one way might be through being open with the child and creating an atmosphere in which the stammer and feelings connected with it can be talked about in an easy manner. After all, if our child is ill, or has been upset by something that has happened, we do not ignore it in the hope that it will 'go away'. Instead, we try to understand what the child is telling us by his words or behaviour. Our feeling is that stammering can be treated in much the same way. We will discuss this more in the next chapter.

(2) Although we have outlined a number of factors which *may* occur at this stage, it is important to reiterate that they are not all seen in all children. Some show only one or two of the features, for example, whilst others demonstrate several but only mildly.

(3) It might seem from the way we have described borderline stammering that it is an all or nothing stage. The child is in it or he is not in it. In reality at this stage there is often very little consistency in the behaviours; one day the child struggles over a word, experiences obvious frustration or even avoids saying something, whereas another day he stammers openly with little struggle and with no concern. In fact, in terms of our three-stage model, the child can drift back and forth for some months, or even longer, between the stages of early dysfluency and borderline stammering.

(4) If borderline stammering is seen as a transition stage from early dysfluency, we might assume that a progression to another stage is inevitable. This, as we will see, is not necessarily the case. With and without professional help, children can and do reduce the hidden part of their dysfluency, return to a stage where it does not concern them greatly or even cease stammering altogether.

Confirmed stammering

To any parent or carer, the words 'confirmed stammering' can understandably paint a very bleak picture. They give the impression of a step having been taken from which there is no turning back. While we do not wish to underestimate the severity of this stage in the development of stammering, we do want to offer some reassurance that things may not be as final and fixed as they sound. Confirmed stammering does not have to be a point of no return.

So once again we ask the question: what do these words mean? Really, the key is in the child's own feelings and beliefs about his stammer. The confirmed stammerer has in fact confirmed himself. He has decided that stammering is not something he *does* but something he *is*. He sees himself first and foremost as a stammerer, not a person who happens to stammer. This can be quite a difficult concept to get hold of, so let us try to explain it more closely. Imagine you are wearing a pair of glasses which distort your vision. Everything you see is affected by the distortion, so things appear differently from the way they once did. When you think about a situation you begin to imagine how it will look through the glasses. You think about how you will behave with the glasses on. Will you walk more carefully, take smaller steps, stay in one small area or might it even be too difficult for you to go into the situation at all? Will you try to pretend that nothing has changed, that you are not really wearing the glasses, even though you are behaving differently from the way you would without them on? Similarly, the confirmed stammerer sees words, situations, people, events wearing his own special glasses. He alters his behaviour accordingly. He tries to hide his stammer, to avoid things which might make others aware of his problem. In fact he tries to present himself as a fluent speaker but his attempts to do so actually make him more of a stammerer.

Let us now look at some fictitious examples of some young people with confirmed stammers.

CONFIRMED CALVIN

Calvin is 15. He is very musical, a member of a steel band and the main 'rap' singer in a group. When he's rapping he is always fluent, he can really express his feelings and it makes him feel very confident. He just wishes it were the same all the time. Sometimes he just can't get the words out at all. He feels he is going to explode sometimes because of all the tension in his body when he speaks. His friends find it very strange that in some situations he talks like everyone else and in others he doesn't seem to be able to string two words together. It is often such an effort when he talks that he just gives up. He doesn't talk about how he feels and no one likes to ask him about his stammer because they don't want to upset him. At school he seems quite shy and never puts his hand up to answer questions. If the teacher asks him a question directly and he thinks he might stammer he pretends not to know the answer. He would prefer that other people think other negative things about him rather than admit that he stammers.

CONFIRMED CAROLINE

Caroline is 11. Her overt stammer varies a lot. Sometimes it is really severe with a great deal of tension, and at other times it is barely noticeable. It is worse when she is with new people. She doesn't have many close friends. Her best friend gets a bit fed up with her when she won't come round to her house and never phones her up. When she asks why, Caroline says she forgot or couldn't be bothered and her friend gets quite upset. Really it's because those are the times she stammers most but she daren't risk telling her friend that. What would she think of her? Her mum complains that she is always up in her room, listening to the radio or playing on the computer. When she asks Caroline why she doesn't come down with the family, Caroline just shrugs her shoulders. At school they have no complaints about her. Her last report described her as a model pupil, always doing as she is told, handing her homework in on time, a hard worker and never any bother.

CONFIRMED CHRIS

Chris is 16, a good-looking young man who is very concerned, like many teenagers, about his image. He wants to wear all the latest gear but finds the things he wants to buy really expensive. He'd like to get a Saturday job so he could finance himself. He hasn't actually applied for any jobs as he doesn't think he has a chance of getting one. Not only is there a lot of competition, which makes his chances slim, but also he doesn't think he could cope with serving people in a shop. How would he manage if he really had to say a word he knew he would stammer on and couldn't change it? It would be no good saying something was 20 pence when it was in fact 19. Most people have no idea that he has a speech problem and he's determined to keep it this way. He usually manages to hide it very well, although he would admit (to himself at least) that there have been some disadvantages in doing this. For example, he is actually very good at French and would have probably got a high exam mark had he taken it as an option. However, he knew it would require a lot of oral work and he just couldn't risk people finding out about his stammer. Recently, he plucked up courage to ask a girl out. When she turned him down he was sure it was because of his stammer – who would want to go out with someone who talked like he did?

You will notice that none of the features with which these young people present are really very different from those occurring at the borderline stage; it is rather that they may be more severe or that there may be more features apparent at this stage.

Features of confirmed stammering

Hiding the stammer and true feelings about stammering We have already spoken of how it is the person's attitudes to the stammer which are the most important feature of this developmental stage. The change in attitude is reflected in behaviour. Some of these will already have been described in the section on borderline stammering. Once again it is often the number or extent of the behaviours which alters in confirmed stammering. Any of the following can occur:

- Intense feelings about the stammer (anger, embarrassment, etc.) which are often kept inside and not spoken about. Sometimes these feelings are denied, even to the person themselves, who develops a 'don't care' attitude. Often at this stage there comes a feeling of resignation. Having stammered for as long as they can remember, they begin to believe that nothing can change, that it will always be the same.
- Avoidance of all manner of things which if confronted risk 'exposing' the stammer. The list of avoidances is infinite but includes such things as specific sounds, words, situations, the expression of emotions, making friends, talking about stammering.
- 'Pretence' – sometimes the young person tries to pretend that the problem is something other than the stammer. He may, for example, pretend to forget his reading book at school, that he doesn't know an answer, that he has forgotten the name of a film star. This type of hiding can become very sophisticated. Hussein, for example, would sometimes respond willingly in class when he knew he could say the word but when he anticipated difficulty, he would don a frown and pretend he didn't know the answer. None of his teachers had any idea that he stammered because his acting was so convincing.
- The development of more solitary pursuits. The former chatterbox may withdraw into record playing or computer games in the privacy of his own room, or spend hours in front of the television.
- Letting others make assumptions. Perhaps one of the most concerning things about this stage of stammering is that often the young person prefers other people to think all manner of things about him, rather than know he has a stammer. Calvin let his teacher and classmates think he didn't know the answer. Caroline allowed her best friend to

think she didn't care enough to contact her. Others choose to let people assume they are shy, indecisive, unintelligent, boring, and so on. Even when others do know that the person stammers, this sort of behaviour is often still apparent. This was brought home to us with one of our clients, Patrick, aged 14, who was passionately interested in pop music. He was being asked by one of us to name five things in a category – five pop groups, five records, five pop singers. He would start to speak, freeze, start again and then say 'I don't know' or 'I've forgotten'. When challenged, he eventually admitted that he did, of course, know all the answers but felt unable to say so or to risk stammering, even though we had spent many sessions talking openly about his stammer.

The overt stammer In confirmed stammering the stammering behaviour may be more severe, or be thought by the person concerned to be more severe. Complete stoppages of sound (blocks) may be apparent and can last for several seconds. Repetitions are sometimes multiple; the person repeats the sound, word or phrase many times. A sound is sometimes stretched out or extended until he runs out of breath and then starts again. However, the overt speech of the person with a confirmed stammer might not be severe at all, in fact he may rarely, if ever, be heard to stammer (as in the case of Chris). This is one of the major difficulties in assessing how severe a person's stammer is; what it *sounds* like is only one part of a much bigger picture. Sometimes avoidance of words, although not necessarily obvious, can make the person's speech sound 'odd' or over-complex. Suzanne found it hard to say 'Saturday', and instead said 'the first day of the weekend' or 'the day after Friday'. Francis sounded as if he was never going to get to the point – he spent so much time 'going round the houses' to avoid the feared word. Gareth got on people's nerves because he often prefaced what he was going to say with 'what I mean to say is' because this 'run in' gave him a lead into saying what he really wanted.

The amount of tension in the stammer One of the features of this stage of stammering is that there is a great deal of tension involved in stammering. This is the case with Calvin who feels as if he might burst with tension. Often the tension is apparent to the listener. This may be seen as a general phenomenon all through the body, or it can be specific to particular areas, such as the mouth, throat or chest. Sometimes it is very obvious, lips are pushed tightly together, fists clenched, veins in the neck stand up. Sometimes it is not visible but experienced internally by the young person. Sometimes it has become such a habit that he does not realize it is there. It is only when it is pointed out, or when the individual has the opportunity to feel what it is like to be relaxed, that the tension is actually noticed.

Uncontrolled breathing patterns Sometimes people who stammer develop very poor patterns of breathing. Some breathe involving only the upper part of their chest and so never take in enough air to be able to continue speaking for more than a few seconds at a time. Others take far too many breaths or not enough. Yet others try to speak when they are breathing in, rather than when they are breathing out.

Increase in extra sounds, words or bodily movements In the section on borderline stammering, we discussed how some of these extra behaviours become incorporated into the stammer. In confirmed stammering, this sort of behaviour may increase in amount and/or in intensity.

Blaming poor performance on stammering Sometimes we find that the young person feels so badly about himself because he stammers he starts to blame failures in other areas of his life on his speech, rather than consider if there might be another reason. Chloë, for example, felt she would be the best in her English group if she could only read fluently, despite her very average ability in the subject. The young person may not be prepared to consider that there may be something other than the stammer to blame when things go wrong. When Calvin was rejected by a girl, his immediate reaction was to blame his stammer (even though he hid it so effectively that it was highly unlikely she even knew about it).

Confirmed stammering and adolescence

Although, as we have said, we do not feel that any stage of stammering is restricted to a particular age range, it is often the case that confirmed stammering occurs in adolescence. This makes our task even more difficult when we try to understand the meaning of some of the behaviours the young person displays. If we look back at our own teenage years, many of us experienced turbulent and traumatic times on our journey into adulthood. For the child there are so many changes happening. Firstly there are the physical or bodily changes which occur. These are often accompanied by anxieties in the young person as to whether they are 'late' or 'early' when these happen, even though there is an enormous variation within the 'normal' range. Then there are the emotional upheavals as young people develop a sense of their own identity and may reject much of what they had previously held to be important. Many parents consider this period a very difficult one to cope with and at times find the person they are dealing with becomes the very opposite of the one they used to know. The once fun-loving extrovert who never seemed to have a care in the world becomes sullen and introverted; the easy-going, thoughtful, caring child becomes moody and flies off the handle for no apparent reason. Difficult times for all! Add to this the traumas of having to contend with a stammer and it is easy to see why this is such a crucial time for the young person who stammers. One of the problems for parents and others is that it can seem almost impossible to try to separate the effects of adolescence from the effects of stammering. Is the child, for example, becoming withdrawn because of the stammer or because he is worried as to whether he is acceptable to his age group for other reasons? Are his mood swings connected to an imbalance in his hormonal system or are they rather a reaction to a lack of self worth he feels because of his stammer? Parents and others need a great deal of patience and understanding at this time to help minimize the effect that the stammer may begin to have at such a time.

5

How parents can help

As we start to write this chapter, we find ourselves considering what to say in the light of what has already been said in the first four chapters, related to the understanding of dysfluency. This, of course, presupposes that readers have actually read them! Whilst some have no doubt done so, our guess is there are others who have chosen to start reading at this chapter. As parents ourselves, we know that when we are concerned about our children, it is what we can *do* to help that interests us most. We would therefore probably have been very tempted to start here ourselves! However, as the saying (nearly) goes, 'Don't do as we do, do as we say'! We would urge readers who have indeed opened the book for the first time here to be patient and return to the beginning. Understanding a problem is, after all, an essential part of dealing with it. If a child, for example, has difficulty in reading, his carer's approach to helping him would depend on the reason for his problem and might be very different if it were because of dyslexia rather than because he was being teased at school. Although, as we have already discussed, one of the frustrations about stammering is that we do not know what causes it, we do have ideas about the factors which are involved and these are discussed in some detail in those earlier chapters.

This chapter is entitled 'How parents can help'. Understandably, as a parent reading the book you might expect to find practical ideas here, perhaps in the form of do's and don'ts, specifying all the useful and not so useful ways of behaving in order to help your child. Had this book been on another subject, such as teaching your child to swim, this kind of advice would have been possible. In fact, in the past, advice given by some speech and language therapists has been predominantly in that kind of format. However, we no longer feel that such an approach is possible in most cases, and particularly in a book such as this which is likely to be read by a wide range of people with differing needs. In addition, we have no crystal ball to tell us which children will grow out of their stammering and which will become fluent. We are able to help parents consider issues and point them towards ideas which can aid the development of fluency, but the child may continue to stammer. It seems to us more important therefore that parents are enabled to do all they can to ensure that their child feels good about himself, whether or not he stammers. In this way, whatever the future brings in terms of fluency or stammering, the individual's choices in life are restricted as little as possible by his speech.

We have therefore divided the chapter into two sections. The first is concerned with feelings, beliefs and attitudes of parents and children about dysfluency which lay the foundation for the way they behave. In order to see whether and how behaviour can be changed, we therefore believe we need first to look at what underlies it. Let us take some examples. Parent A believes that stammering is something his child does deliberately in order to seek attention. His behaviour might therefore involve some form of punishment, such as telling the child off when he stammers. Parent B feels sorry for her child when he stammers. Her behaviour, as a consequence, involves indulging the child and rarely telling him off. The second section in this chapter is more practical and offers ideas as to when and how behaviours can be changed. Some of these changes may lead to alterations in the child's communication and an increase in fluency. Other changes are not to be directed specifically towards speech but aim to foster the child's positive self-esteem and ensure that the stammer does not have as great an impact on him. It can be that such an approach also indirectly increases fluency: because the child feels better about himself, his stammer takes on less significance and he stammers less.

Recognize your own feelings

Over the years we have become aware of just how many and how varied are the emotions which parents and carers experience. As you read through just some of the feelings we have heard expressed, consider which of them you have felt yourself.

Guilt

This seems to be an almost inevitable part of child rearing. When something happens that makes us unhappy, concerned or worried, how many times do we feel we must be to blame? Often this feeling of guilt is made worse if we have a similar problem to the child's – we are short, have thin hair or a temptation for sweet foods, and so on. If a parent stammers they may well feel their child's stammer is because of them. Indeed we have known many adult clients who have delayed or even put off having children because they are afraid that their offspring will develop the same problem. (Interestingly, parents are not so likely to take responsibility when their child shows a particular talent or does well in something. They are more likely then to say 'I don't know where he gets it from, it's not me!') Sometimes the guilt which is felt is reinforced by the comments of others. Perhaps the parents have been told that the child will 'grow out' of the stammer but he has not, so the parents feel they must be to blame. Maybe they think they should have sought professional help earlier. People will often give well-meaning but not always useful advice as to how parents should handle the problem. When the parents do not follow the advice and the stammer remains, they imagine that others are saying 'I told you so'. In our experience, parents often link their child's stammer to a particular event (such as moving house) or emotional trauma (such as parents' separation).

There are a couple of things about guilt when related to stammering which we feel are worth mentioning. First of all we would refer you back to the earlier chapters of the book. The evidence we have does not point to any one cause for stammering – it is likely to involve a number of factors. There is, however, evidence that parents can be helpful in maximizing their child's potential for fluency. Secondly, guilt is not constructive: it doesn't actually help or change anything. We can waste a lot of time, with hindsight, telling ourselves 'If only I had done this or that'. However, we cannot change what has happened. We can look at what we might do *now*.

Anger

Often when something is 'wrong' with our child we feel angry. We may feel a great sense of injustice and ask ourselves 'Why my child?' When that question cannot fully be answered we feel even more angry. The anger is often projected onto others. In the case of the dysfluent child it is sometimes directed to another family member, perhaps someone who shows less patience that we think they should, to someone else in the family or in the neighbourhood who stammers, to another child who brought the stammer to our child's attention, intentionally or unintentionally. Often we blame ourselves, particular people, or society in general, in order to try to make sense of the problem or to give our anger a focus. In our own families, we are aware that it is all too easy for us to blame someone who has hurt our child in some way, rather than face up to the fact that maybe our child provoked the reaction by his or her own behaviour. Perhaps we need to ask ourselves whether our anger, justified or not, is actually helping the child to deal with the problem. If not, we need to seek alternatives that are more constructive.

Loss of ideals

Parents-to-be are often asked if they want a boy or a girl. The answer many people give is 'I really don't mind as long as it's all right'. Whilst this is the main concern of most parents, it is natural to fantasize about the sort of child we might have – boy or girl, blonde or brunette, tall or short. We may also project our fantasies into the future – will the child be a basketball player, a singer, a doctor, a linguist? When the child turns out (like all children) not to be 'perfect', and is too short, tone-deaf, hates science or French, we may have to revise our ambitions. If he has a stammer, do we hold on to our dreams, do we revise them in terms of the child as a whole, or do we see the stammer as a restriction of our own and our child's ambitions?

Pain

It is never easy to see our children suffering in any way. When our babies cry or our children are upset, we seem almost to be programmed to respond and help them. We often feel the need to take the pain away. Sometimes we can do this. We can feed the baby, change his nappy, give him a cuddle. When the young child falls over, we put a plaster on the cut and 'kiss it better'. When he is ill we take him to the doctor and give him his medicine. If the child is hurt in other ways, it is often less easy to help. We cannot protect our children from being hurt emotionally – it is part of the growing process. The child who stammers, like the child who is fat, thin, spotty, bad at sport has ultimately to learn to cope with his difficulties himself. We can try to help him to cope better, talk over his difficulties, modify the stresses in his environment but we cannot take his problem away, however much we wish. For those parents who desperately want to protect their child, this can be hard to come to terms with.

Embarrassment

Parents may be embarrassed about stammering in a number of ways.

- Frequently they tell us that they are embarrassed for their child. They watch other people listening to them, see them react in a negative way, and 'feel for' the child.
- Sometimes parents feel embarrassed for the listener who doesn't seem to know what to do when the child stammers.
- Parents understandably sometimes feel embarrassed for themselves. They wonder what others are thinking and whether they are devaluing the child or the parent because of the way the child talks.

These feelings of embarrassment often occur because of a lack of communication or understanding. The parent does not know what the child or listener is actually feeling and so imagines the worst. The listener doesn't know how to react and senses that the parent does not want them to notice the dysfluency and is left not knowing how best to behave.

Worry

What parent does not worry about their child? We worry about all manner of things from the moment the child is born – or before! Often our worry is directed to the future: we are concerned about what will happen if. . . . Relating this to stammering, parents ask 'what will happen if he stammers at nursery, at primary school, at high school, at university, at work? Will he be teased, overlooked, undervalued? Will he make friends, find a partner? Will he always stammer, will it get worse or better?' While we understand how urgent the need for answers to these questions can feel, we think it is important to try and stay with how things are *here and now*. The questions are, in any case, unanswerable. We do not know what the future will bring, there is no crystal ball we can refer to which will answer our questions. Worrying about the future does not change anything but there are other things which can be done which might.

Recognize what your child is feeling

What we are talking about here is really the development of empathy. The word empathy means 'feeling into'. If we are empathic towards a child we understand what things are like from his perspective, rather than imposing our own understanding on the child. Let us take an example. A child is watching a television programme. To us, through our adult eyes, the programme is boring, unrealistic and meaningless. It neither informs nor entertains us. What of the child? He feels quite differently. To him it is exciting and stimulating. It allows him to escape, to dream, to identify with his heroes and imagine himself carrying out some of their fearless pursuits. Now let us turn to stammering. Is our perception the same as the child's? Take a child at the early dysfluent stage. Three-year-old Mary is telling her Auntie about her morning at playgroup. As her parents watch her taking a long time to get the words out they experience a whole range of emotions such as annoyance, frustration, embarrassment and upset, and assume Mary is feeling these too. In reality she probably has no awareness that her speech is any different from that of other people. If she does react at all negatively it is probably just with a mild and momentary frustration when she is not able to say what she wants to as quickly as she would like. Of course, it is also easy to underestimate the child's feelings. Mark, who is 15, tells his parents something and speaks fairly fluently. They notice a small amount of hesitation and perhaps are aware that he doesn't look at them when he talks. They assume he is feeling generally OK about his communication, perhaps just a little preoccupied. In reality, he is picking and choosing his words to find those which are easiest to say. He is looking away because he is intensely embarrassed and doesn't want to risk seeing similar feelings on their faces.

If we are able to see the dysfluency as the child sees it, we are more able to help him to deal with it. When the child is not aware of his dysfluency or is aware but does not see it as a problem, then we might ask ourselves if it is actually a problem at all. If, however, it is seen as a problem by the child we need to know what sort of difficulty is being experienced in order that we can help.

How to help

So, having looked at how the child feels and whether this is the same or different from how we feel, what happens next? What can parents and carers actually do? Now we want to look at some practical steps parents can take to help their child. We do not know if this help will result in the child becoming more fluent. Sometimes it will. Hopefully, it will always help in sustaining or increasing the child's feeling of wellbeing or self-esteem so that he feels better about himself, whether or not he stammers.

The ideas we present are inevitably very general. Some you will find to be appropriate for your child or your family, others not. Some may be easy to employ and others difficult or impossible. It is important to remember that perfect parents do not exist. We are all human. We usually do the best we can at the time, according to the circumstances we find ourselves in. That is the most we can ever hope to do.

Help the child feel good about himself and his talking

We have already discussed how, as stammering develops, the child can become more concerned about his speech until eventually he sees his identity as a stammerer rather than someone who stammers. Parents may be able to help stop or slow down this process, and the following ideas are useful.

Try to listen to what your child is saying, rather than to how he is saying it In this way you will probably find you enjoy conversations more and your child will feel that his thoughts and ideas are valued. If you look at him and respond to what he says with interest he will be more likely to find communication pleasant. If you direct your concentration to the content of your child's speech, you are also less likely to show negative reactions to his dysfluency. Sometimes parents are not aware of displaying these reactions, which can be very subtle. Brian's dad, for example, stiffens slightly when his son stammers and then relaxes when he is fluent again. Nasim's mum looks away for just a split second when her daughter is dysfluent. Sometimes people are aware of these responses but find them difficult to alter. Perhaps you might recognize some of them in yourself or others. It is often hard not to show your feelings if you are concerned. It is sometimes surprising how sensitive some young children are to even the smallest of reactions. Concentrating on the *what* rather than the *how* of what is being said sometimes helps reduce these behaviours and, consequently, negative messages about his speaking are not relayed to the child.

Build a relationship with the child in which he feels able to talk about any problems he is experiencing Try to ensure that the child feels able to tell you of his worries and concerns if he wants to. It is all too easy for a 'conspiracy of silence' to develop over stammering. Many of our adult clients tell us that as children they felt unable to talk about stammering with their parents because it was never mentioned, as if it were something to be ashamed of. They say they would have liked to have been more able to talk about how they were feeling but somehow saw it as a taboo subject. However, deciding when and how to talk about stammering is by no means easy. Let us consider the developmental stages of stammering:

- The child at the early dysfluent stage is generally unaware or, for the most part at least, unconcerned about his dysfluency. We do not, of course, want to risk making him concerned about his speech. Much of the time all that is required is for the parent just to listen to the child patiently and wait for him to complete what he is saying without commenting. However, that is not to say we should always ignore it or pretend nothing is happening. Instead it is possible to acknowledge temporary frustrations, in much the same way as we might comfort a child who stumbles as he starts to walk. As we have already discussed, the process of learning to talk is a complex one. Letting the child know we understand that it is sometimes difficult to say all that he wants, in the way he wants, when he wants, can be very reassuring at times. Let us look at an example. Joanna, aged 5, runs to tell her mum that she has just seen her friend's car draw up outside. She is going to a pantomime with the friend and is very excited. She reaches the word 'car' but says it over and over, eventually stamping her foot and sighing with frustration. Her mum looks at her while she talks, shows she is interested and has time to listen. She may also add something along the lines of 'It can be really hard to say things sometimes when we are excited, can't it?'

- The child whose dysfluency is at the borderline stage has some idea that there is something different about the way he talks and may make some attempt to disguise or hide it. If we are willing to discuss stammering with him, show him we understand how frustrating it can be, want to help and still value his contribution as much as if he did not stammer, he is likely to be less inclined to hide his dysfluency. Qasim, for example, starts to tell his dad about a football match. He gets stuck on a few words and his dad notices he is changing some of them. He tells him 'You seem to be changing some of the words in case you get stuck. You know, I'm really much more interested to hear all the details of the match, just tell me all about it. I've plenty of time to wait if you get stuck.'

- The child at the confirmed stammering stage feels bad about stammering. He needs to know he can have a safe haven in which to share his fears, embarrassment, anger and so on with those who care for him. If the stammer is never mentioned, he may begin to believe (as one of our clients told us she did), that it is too awful for his parents to mention. It may help to acknowledge moments of struggle ('That sounded really hard for you to say') or ask how the child feels about something and help him to plan strategies ('Would it help to tell Mr Jones that you are worried about stammering before you give your talk?'). In this way the problems associated with the stammer are shared and the burden the child carries does not feel so heavy.

Although we have said that the channels of communication about stammering should be kept open, we do not wish to imply that parents should forever be discussing their child's speech! We do not want the child to feel that the way in which he talks matters most. In fact the reverse is true. Rather we need to ensure stammering is something which can be talked about when appropriate so that the child feels it remains something he does rather than something he is.

Value the child as he is, not as you might want him to be Most of us want the very best for our children and are disappointed if we feel that something like a stammer could prevent them from achieving their potential. However, we only need to look to some of the famous people in this century to see that stammering does not have to be a bar in any field. Marilyn Monroe, King George VI, Winston Churchill, Bruce Willis are all examples of people who stammered but still made it in their chosen field. A child of one of the authors struggled academically at school. Initially it was hard for her parents to see her falling behind her peers and feeling a sense of failure. The situation changed for the better when she started at a new school. Here she was valued as a person in her own right, regardless of her academic abilities. She became more positive about herself generally and began to take pride in her work and as she did so her achievements increased too. As parents we also started to realize it was because of her struggle that she had developed a sensitive and caring side of her nature. Had she not had those difficulties, she might have been a very different person. We are not trying to suggest that stammering is to be welcomed but rather we would say that if it is accepted, the child not only is more likely to feel good about himself but may also be more likely to increase his fluency.

Remember the scales, find out what helps them balance

The fluency of many children is robust and not easily upset by increased demands. Some children, however, react to these by becoming dysfluent. Try to identify the weights (demands) which seem to upset the balance for your own child. Here is a list of things which parents we have known have identified as useful to consider. Remember as you look through it that the list will be different for each child and it is only the *balance* we are trying to adjust. We are not aiming for perfection, we are all human after all.

Demands which can affect the child's fluency

Questions Adults tend to ask children a lot of questions as one of the main ways of finding out what they want to know. If our children have been at school, for example, we understandably want to find out what has happened while they have been away. Depending on their age we ask such things as:

- What did you do?
- What did you have for dinner?
- Why didn't you eat your apple?
- Who did you play with?
- Have you got any homework?
- When are you going to phone Nana?

Often we ask one question after another, hardly giving the child time to draw breath after one before we come in with the next! While this way of communicating is perfectly natural and most children are able (if not always willing!) to respond without difficulty, it can put pressure on a child, particularly a young one, to speak when he might not particularly want to or feels he has nothing to say. It also demands a certain form of reply containing specific information within a given time limit. This may consequently affect the child's fluency on some occasions. It can, therefore, be helpful to rephrase some of our questions as statements. If we look at those questions we have used as illustrations we might instead say:

- I wonder what you've been doing today.
- You had football this morning – I bet you were ready for your dinner.
- I see you haven't eaten your apple.
- I saw Sue today at work. I suppose you played with Joe.
- Wednesday is usually homework day, so I guess you've brought some home.
- Perhaps we can work out when you've time to phone Nana.

This kind of approach allows the child some freedom in their response and its timing. Having more control can in turn help fluency.

Demanding speech Asking a child to speak can put pressure on some children in much the same way that asking questions does. The sort of things we are thinking of here are the following (heard in almost all households from dawn to dusk!):

- Say thank-you to Auntie Eileen.
- Tell your Dad what happened at school.
- Say that poem you learned at school.

Once again, a specific set of words is required at a set time. In some situations there is additional pressure such as a number of people listening and looking or a fear of getting it wrong. While most children deal with these demands with no difficulty (and if they didn't most of the population would be dysfluent, we do so much of it) there are some children in whom the result may be a breakdown of fluency. If this is the case with your child it may help to experiment with reducing this kind of communicative pressure. Instead of telling the child what to say, allow him to decide what he wants to say and when (at least within reason!). Let us look at possible alternatives to the responses above. In reply to Auntie Eileen's gift, the child may give her a kiss, send a letter or thank her verbally at a time of his own choosing (perhaps when they are alone together without an audience). Dad may have to wait to hear what happened at school or mum will have to tell him herself if it is she who wants him to know. The poem might remain unsaid for the time being.

Interruptions and not feeling able to interrupt Young children in particular often feel a tremendous urgency in what they want to say. While the content may not seem important to the adult, the young child has a great desire to share his thoughts as they come into his head, without filtering them according to audience interest or relevance to the situation. In addition, children quite easily forget what they are saying if they have to hold it in their heads for too long. If they are unable to interrupt, not only do they lose interest in what they are going to say but they can lose track of their thoughts and stumble over their words when their turn does finally come. It is quite difficult to allow children to interrupt adults, even if this does seem to help enhance their fluency. Parents we have known have found it helpful to explain to other family and friends just why they are letting this happen. They might say 'Samantha finds it difficult to hold on to her ideas for very long and it seems to make it easier for her to speak if we let her interrupt us when possible'. In this way it enables other people to be more tolerant when they are required to stop what they are saying and allow the child to interrupt them.

Research has shown that people interrupt children more often when their speech is dysfluent than when it is fluent. Sometimes this is to give advice, sometimes to fill in words when they are hard to say. It is interesting to note, however, that if children are interrupted when they are speaking, they can find speech control hard to re-establish when their turn is given back. Given time, patience and an attentive audience, children can usually say the things they want to.

Adults talking too fast It may be that when children listen to adults who speak quickly, they feel a need to reply at a similar rate. This rate might be too fast for the young child who is not able to co-ordinate his thoughts or his muscles at speed. If the adult slows his rate of speaking, he is providing a good model for the child to copy. The child is then more likely to respond similarly and thus has more time to synchronize his ideas with the movements needed for speech.

Time pressure There are two main kinds of time pressure which can have a bearing on a child's fluency. The first concerns the pressure for the child to answer within time limits. We have already looked at how asking questions or demanding speech or particular kinds of speech can be difficult for the dysfluent child. Then there is the general rush and busyness which is apparent in many households. We touched on this in Chapter 3. It is important that the child feels there is time to consider what he has to say and how to say it, and that his remarks do not have to be squeezed in between other things. Sometimes it is helpful to establish a 'special time' just for child and parent in which they do something enjoyable together which involves talking. If it is hard to find this time, it can be an indication of how little time the family has available for talking. However, there is only some point in doing this if it is something which is pleasurable for the child. We suggested this to a mother and initially it worked well. Then one day the nine-year-old child said to her 'Do you mind if we don't have our special time today? I'd just like to go and listen to music in my room'. This serves as a reminder to us that some children need space as well as time. They may benefit from a quiet time, perhaps in a room on their own, where they might sit with a book, listen to music, watch television – in fact do not have to talk at all.

Turn taking We have mentioned that children sometimes find it harder to speak fluently when they fear being interrupted. Some also experience difficulties when they have problems establishing their turn. This can be an issue in large families or where there are articulate members who have a lot to say or who are older and able to speak at a more rapid rate and turns pass quickly from one to another. Timing is of the essence in such situations, and if young Susie doesn't manage to initiate her message in a slight gap in the conversation there is always someone ready to take over. Establishing turns and helping family members feel they have a right to be heard is important for all families but needs particular attention in a family where one member is dysfluent.

Language and cultural issues Some children have an additional demand on them which can be one factor in tipping the scales towards dysfluency. These are children who speak two languages. Many children cope with an additional language without difficulty and indeed relish the richness this brings to their lives. Others find it more of a problem and it is one factor in their speech becoming dysfluent. This is perhaps because the demand of an extra language acts as a sort of overload on the child's overall language development system. In addition, some children face extra demands because of their culture or religion: they have to study and read particular books, perhaps in yet another language or learn passages from scripture. Again, whilst the majority will find this stimulating and cope without difficulty, for others it is an additional pressure. Often things settle down once the child has reached a certain level of competence in both languages. However, it may be that some other demands need to be reduced for these children who have more than one language to contend with.

Other issues to consider

The following are factors which we have found over the years to be important ones in *some* families. We do not suggest that they are all relevant to all families but rather that they *may* be useful points to consider as you go about the task of trying to help your dysfluent child.

Coping with excitement

The speech of many young children is more dysfluent when they are excited. Children vary in their ability to cope with excitement. Some manage it easily and find the events an enriching part of their lives. Others appear to react adversely, especially when high levels are maintained. We are aware, for example, that our own children's behaviour when young was often diabolical at their birthdays. It sometimes felt like a very poor reward for the hours of effort we put into making the occasion memorable! For some dysfluent children it seems to be helpful either to endeavour to keep excitement levels low or to help the child to manage excitement better. You may find some of the following ideas helpful:

- Giving forewarning and 'preparing' the child for the exciting activity if this seems to help. For example, telling him what will happen, who will be there, what he will do, etc. Some children find that if they know the ropes, they gain a feeling of control, others seem to cope best when they do not anticipate things before they happen.
- Spacing exciting activities where possible.
- Planning for 'recovery' times where nothing much is happening and relaxation can ensue.
- Introducing only one exciting idea or activity at a time (for example, telling the child that they are going to the seaside at the weekend but not mentioning a planned trip to the cinema the following day).
- Talking about the proposed event in a calm way, rather than in a way which is more likely to over-stimulate the child.
- Trying to ensure the child gets enough rest and sleep at these times.

Giving advice

As parents, we are always giving advice to our children and indeed they often seek it from us. We can use our experience to aid their development and help them to cope more effectively with their lives. There are times, however, when we know that our children have to find their own solutions, for a number of reasons:

- We don't have the answer! We may, however, be able to help the child find it (for example, by consulting an encyclopaedia, seeing the doctor, asking the teacher and so on, depending on the nature of the problem).
- We don't fully understand the problem. We see it in one way, the child sees it in another. The child, for example, says that he is no good at

football. He is in the school team so we find this hard to believe. However, he knows that he is only just good enough to keep his place and risks being dropped in future matches.

- Our answer is not appropriate for the child. Our answer to our teenage daughter who is feeling cold might be for her to put on a vest or an extra jumper but this is not even considered by her – it would ruin her 'street credibility'. It is worth remembering that so often when we say 'If I were you', what we really mean is 'If you were me'!

- If we always supply the answers, the child does not learn to solve his own problems and may always look to others when problems arise. If we approach difficulties jointly, however, helping them to explore possible options and come to their own conclusions, we are laying a foundation for more effective coping in the future.

How does this apply to stammering? It is sometimes all too easy to provide an answer, without understanding the problem or seeing some of the possible implications of our answers. Let us take a couple of examples. Martha, aged 6, stammers and also speaks very quickly. Her parents tell her to speak more slowly and indeed she is often more fluent when she does so. Seemingly a useful strategy but there are other factors which have not been taken into account. Martha is unaware of any problems in speaking. If she is told frequently to slow down, she is likely to start to believe that perhaps there is something wrong with the way she speaks and also that others pay more attention to *how* she says things than to *what* she says. She tries out her parents' suggestion but finds it too difficult to think about speech rate as well the ideas she is trying to express. She may then try other ways of putting her speech right – she starts to struggle as she does so or avoids expressing her ideas on occasions if she feels they will not be fully listened to. Our second example involves Joe, aged 14. He hides his stammer very effectively by changing words on which he anticipates having difficulty. In this way he appears very fluent. His parents have seen this happen on occasions. They mention that it seems to be helping him and suggest he does it more often. It could be seen as a useful strategy as Joe's fluency has increased over the past months. Of course, what is actually happening is that Joe's stammering is getting worse. Not the overt, obvious part but the covert, hidden part. Joe is now beginning to see his stammer as something which is bad and to be covered up.

Protecting the child

As parents we have a wholly understandable desire to protect our children from being hurt. We are incensed if we learn they have been injured, mentally or physically, by others and sometimes feel the need to intervene. Often this is totally appropriate, especially with younger children who do not have the skills to deal with these things themselves. At other times, as we have discussed, the child needs help to 'fight his own battles' and even to find his own solutions (which may not be those we would have chosen for him). Sometimes our reaction to our child's hurt is to wrap him metaphorically in cotton wool, to try to protect him from any possible upset. As children grow older, they have gradually to take on more and more independence in order to cope without their parents in adult life. They have, for example, to learn to cross roads, go on buses, find their way around town. The time they are first allowed to do these things will vary according to the child, the parents and the environment, but it will have to happen eventually. When it does, the child inevitably faces risks but we recognize that these risks are part and parcel of growing up. Similarly, the child who stammers has to learn to cope with the reactions of others, imagined or real. As parents we have to be aware of a fine balance between caring for the child and over-protecting them. Some parents find it hard not to speak for their child so that others do not see the stammer. A friend, for example, asks the child a question and the parent immediately jumps in with an answer. The child is not seen to stammer but perhaps this would not have happened anyway. In addition he has not had the opportunity to express his thoughts and ideas. If the stammer is mentioned by others in front of the child, parents sometimes change the conversation so that the child is not upset. Perhaps other alternatives are not considered. Had the comment been addressed a number of things could have occurred: the person might have increased their understanding, and the child might have felt that the stammer was able to be discussed in a matter-of-fact way.

Recognizing the boundaries between helping children to deal better with stammering and over-protecting them is not easy but it is an important area for consideration.

Helping the child to deal with teasing or bullying is another important area. We will discuss this in some detail in the chapter about schools. We would, at this stage, like to recommend some books which deal specifically with this area. *Helping Children Cope with Bullying* by Sarah Lawson, looks at how to recognize when a child is being bullied, why children are bullied or become bullies and how best to help. It offers practical coping strategies and stresses the need to be prepared for bullying, especially if there is something about the child which could make him an easily identifiable target. Our only reservation about the book is that it describes stammering as a sign of anxiety. We would strongly dispute this view which is not based on any research evidence but on an all-too-often held stereotype of stammering. *Don't Pick on Me* by Rosemary Stones also defines bullying and explores different ways of dealing with it. It could be read by older children. There is also an excellent book on the subject of bullying written for children, called *Bully for You* by Toni Goffe. This is described as being a book for bullies or for those who follow bullies. It has eye-catching full-page illustrations and uses humour effectively to illustrate points.

Discipline

Many parents find administering discipline difficult to handle. It is not easy to know how strict or lenient we should be and what sort of punishments or sanctions to apply. It can seem even more difficult if the child becomes more dysfluent when told off. (Sometimes parents feel they cannot tell their child off for this reason. In rare circumstances, if this is the case, it is possible that the child could begin to get emotional 'pay-offs' from stammering – he misbehaves but if he stammers he is less likely to be told off. We are not suggesting that this happens at a conscious level but at a sub-conscious one.)

How is it best to deal with discipline in the dysfluent child? Perhaps we should start by saying that stammering itself should never be the reason for punishment. There is no evidence to suggest that a child might stammer deliberately (apart from a few moments occasionally in imitation, much as he 'tries out' any number of other behaviours, such as accents, funny faces and so on). Neither should stammering be a reason in itself for not disciplining the child. Growing children need to know that there are limits and, if they are not able to stay inside the boundaries themselves, their parents can ensure their safety. Sometimes children understand and acknowledge that these boundaries are necessary, if not at the time then when things have calmed down.

It is helpful, where possible, to use negotiation rather than punishment. Simon, aged 12, wants to watch a video which his parents feel is not suitable for him. He argues that all his friends have seen it and it's *not fair*! Rather than get into a situation where there is a winner and a loser, perhaps it is possible to find a film which both parties are happy with. Penny, aged 15, wants to go to a party and come home with her friends on the bus. Her parents feel this is too dangerous. They are willing to collect her, but Penny can't bear her friends to see her parents. Instead, they negotiate an arrangement whereby Penny and her best friend walk a few metres to the end of the road where the party is held and her parents pick her up there, out of sight of her other friends. In this way no one loses. With younger children, distraction can often prevent a situation becoming too confrontational. The two-year-old starts to pull a plug out of a socket, Mum says a strong 'No!' while finding an interesting toy to keep the child's attention.

Most parents try their best to be fair, reasonable and consistent in their approach to discipline and punishment. However, most of us recognize that we do not always succeed in our endeavours – the way we react is often not based purely on the misdemeanour itself but on our own mood and tolerance level at the time. If we have had a good day, feel well and relaxed, we will hopefully deal with our six-year-old's refusal to go to bed, our eleven-year-old's request for yet another weird T-shirt or our teenager's request to go to an allnight party, in a calm and reasonable manner. If, however, we have had a lousy day, made mistakes at work, forgotten to buy any cat food and argued with our partner, the same situation is likely to be dealt with in a totally different manner. In reality, all we can do is try our best and approach discipline in the context of a loving relationship, recognizing that our child needs a certain degree of security in order to feel safe but also needs some freedom to find his own solutions. Striking a balance is hard.

Significant others

We are aware that children, especially as they get older, are influenced by people outside their immediate family, and these people have quite a bearing on how children learn to see themselves You recall that we discussed this in Chapter 2. In our work, we often explore with parents how to identify and modify factors which seem to have a bearing on the child's developing dysfluency. We then discover that the child actually spends most of his day with a relative or childminder who is unaware of the child's needs in this area. Perhaps, for example, this person always talks over the child or becomes impatient whenever he stammers. Maybe he tells the child to 'stop stammering' or to 'say it properly'. It is important that all who are involved with the child try to work in the same way to help him. In a later chapter we will look at how teachers can help but here we want to consider other carers, relatives and friends. Wherever possible and appropriate, it is sensible to tell other people about your child's dysfluency and the way you are trying to help him, in order to ensure that they take a similar stance. Generally, people are only too pleased to do something to help. If they still react in a way you feel is unhelpful or even harmful, it may be necessary to remind them quite forcefully of how you would like them to behave. If they are unable or unwilling to change, it may, as a last resort, be necessary to review the amount of time the child spends with them.

Other important points

Children are different

Although this point has been made in earlier chapters, we feel it is important enough to be repeated. We do not know why some children stammer and others do not. We do, however, know that children vary considerably in their ability to 'balance the scales'. Some children appear able to take on a multitude of demands while their fluency remains intact. Others react to the smallest of demands with a breakdown in fluency. We have no way of forecasting how children will respond to demands.

Don't feel responsible

In our experience, when parents read or are told about things that may enhance their children's fluency, they often feel very guilty. The immediate response is frequently something along the lines of 'I do that – I interrupt/speak quickly/say 'slow down'/look away – it must be my fault'. We do not think this is the case. Neither do we believe that a child is dysfluent because the *parent* behaves in a particular way. Rather we think that the parent responds in this way because the *child* is dysfluent. However, behaving in an alternative way is likely to give the child the best opportunity to recover from the dysfluency.

Accept the dysfluency

Perhaps the hardest message for a parent to hear is that their child *may* always stammer. While most children recover from stammering, one in a hundred adults stammers. It is easy to see this in a totally negative way, but it does not have to be so. Much will depend on how the individual feels about himself. If he still feels good as a person, his stammer will not have an enormous bearing on his life. We know of many adults who stammer but lead as happy and interesting lives as anyone else – they marry, have children, hold down a good job and so on. Some even become speech and language therapists; indeed in America it seems to be a basic qualification for a specialist in dysfluency! Very often the only restrictions, as with us all, are those the person places on himself. While parents need to understand the problems their child experiences and do all they can to help him increase his fluency, they must also accept the possibility that the child's stammer will not go away. If, in doing this, they prevent the stammer from limiting the child, then they are doing the best they can for their child.

See a speech and language therapist

If you are concerned about your child's speech, seeing a specialist in speech gives you the opportunity to talk over your feelings and discuss helpful approaches for you and your child. It is your right to be seen: don't let anyone put you off!

We hope that after reading this chapter you now understand more about how you have come to feel as you do about your child's dysfluency and will know whether your child feels the same or differently. We have tried also to offer some ideas that, from our experience and from the research which has been undertaken, seem to be helpful in both promoting fluency and ensuring the dysfluent child feels good about himself as a person. In future chapters we will look at how professional workers also help in this process.

6

Getting help

So now you want some help. It may be that as a parent you feel you can no longer manage by yourself. You have tried all the tricks up your sleeve, kept quiet or given all the advice you thought would be useful, listened to friends and neighbours with the same or different problems, and read magazine articles and books until you do not know which way is up. Now you need someone else to advise you on how to help your child.

Perhaps you have reached this point from a different route. It could be that someone else has commented on your child's speech. A teacher or health visitor may have noticed your child having some problems in conversation with them and had a quiet word with you. Now you feel bad that you did not notice the problem yourself, or perhaps angry with 'professional' interference in your parenting.

Whatever the route, you are now looking for outside assistance for your child or a child about whom you care. Where do you go to get that help? It is very difficult to advise people at this point which direction to take, as it is a bit of a 'Catch 22' situation. The steps taken depend largely on the type of help people would find most useful for their circumstances, but individuals will generally find it difficult to decide what is best or most useful until they have tried the various options. Hopefully, reading this chapter will help. What we propose to do in this section is outline the various options that are currently available with details of how to proceed, make contact, get an appointment and so on, in each case. You may then make a more informed choice, know what steps to take and have a better understanding about what you can expect from the 'helper'.

Speech and language therapy

Speech and language therapists are professionally trained and registered individuals (mostly women) who work with children and adults who have difficulties with communication and feeding. Speech and language therapists undergo a three or four year degree training course and are then registered to work in a variety of settings (e.g. hospitals, community clinics, schools and nurseries). The type of situation in which they work often depends upon the kinds of people they wish to help: therapists wishing to specialize in therapy for disabled children will, for example, work in special schools, institutions, day care centres and so on. A few therapists work in independent practice. Their training enables therapists to look at speech problems from a variety of perspectives – they study the medical, linguistic and psychological aspects of a wide range of speech problems, including stammering. Most therapists who go on to specialize in the treatment of stammering have also completed a number of additional courses relating to dysfluency and will be members of a special interest group in this area.

Historically the speech and language therapy profession emerged from the elocutionists of the Victorian era. They developed into a profession in their own right after World War I, with the Royal College of Speech and Language Therapists established in 1945 in London at a time when local authorities were first required to provide education for verbally impaired children. Although often confused with elocutionists and voice teachers, speech and language therapists have no associations at all with these professionals.

Speech therapists have been associated with the treatment of stammering since the very earliest days of their work. Over the years their approach to the treatment of children who stammer has evolved and changed considerably. There has been a noticeable shift of emphasis away from simply teaching a child ways of speaking which hide his dysfluency. (These techniques involved such things as speaking with a rhythmical beat or a regular stress pattern, speaking slowly and rewarding the child for fluent speech.) Currently speech therapists take a more holistic view of the child, as we have discussed in the scales model, examining all the factors which may contribute to the dysfluent speech. You should expect the therapist to talk to you about the history of your child's development, how his speech including the non-fluencies developed, how he gets on in the family, at school and with his peers, and other factors we have discussed in Chapter 2. The therapist may also play with your child or engage him in some other game or activity. This will help to put the child at ease and enables the therapist to hear his speech. It does not matter at this stage whether the child stammers in front of the therapist. She will believe what you report about the child's talking. With young children and those in the early dysfluent stage most of the therapy, if it is required, is carried out indirectly, through the parents, carers, nursery, play group or school staff. A therapist would rarely work directly on a child's speech at this stage. Where the child shows signs of developing a pattern of speech more akin to stammering or is expressing concern himself, then the therapist may work with both the child and the other carers. These days specific exercises which involve teaching the child to alter his normal speech would only be taught in certain circumstances (such as if the therapist believes the child needs to be able to control his dysfluency). These techniques are rarely taught on their own and therapy is also concerned with how an older child thinks of himself as a person and a speaker.

If it is thought that your child would benefit from therapy a variety of regimes are available. Therapy may be on a weekly basis for a certain number of weeks. In some situations you could be asked to bring your child more intensively, perhaps twice or three times a week or daily for a week. In other cases the therapist could ask you to carry out certain tasks at home or work on specific targets. In this instance she is more likely just to keep an eye on your child and monitor his progress periodically, perhaps once per month or every six weeks or even during school holidays and midterm breaks. The quality of therapy should not be measured by the contact the therapist has with the child. The therapist will choose a regime and a frequency of meetings which she believes best suit the needs of your child.

In some cases children are offered therapy with other children in a group. This is not a cheaper alternative to individual therapy but again is an option which the therapist thinks will benefit your child. As communication is an interactive behaviour it makes sense that any therapy used to encourage this among children should be carried out in a natural situation – and a group is just that. Groups are great for getting children talking and working together. They are also useful in therapy as they are the closest we as therapists get to seeing how children communicate with their peers and helping them with this process. Groups also help, encourage and support children. Lucy, an adolescent girl with a stammer, was reluctant to try any of the speech techniques we had worked on in therapy outside with her school friends. We were able to use the group as a safe environment for her to practise these new skills on other peers before tackling the dreaded classroom.

Occasionally parents are given the opportunity to meet other parents in a group situation. They may meet in an adjacent room at the same time as the children have their group or be offered a separate time and venue. In either case the agenda is often set by the parents: they can discuss particular difficulties in coping with dysfluent speech in children, or ask a therapist to provide more information on stammering and the therapy in which their children are involved. Most parents find the opportunity to share their problems and learn more about the management of stammering is time well spent.

Speech and language therapists operate an open referral system. This means that you can contact a therapist directly and ask for an appointment to discuss the child's problems or for the child to be seen.

You may also ask other professionals to send a referral to a speech and language therapist on your behalf. Referrals are accepted from general practitioners, health visitors, teachers and others, but the child would not be seen, for example, in school without the consent of the parents or guardian.

A national directory of therapists is held by the Royal College of Speech and Language Therapists and further details of what is provided in your area can be obtained from them (see Useful addresses section). More local information is usually available from local health services, hospital or community trust headquarters. It would be useful to talk to the speech and language therapy manager or head of service. This person should be able to give you specific information on where your local speech and language therapist or specialist in stammering is based.

We strongly advise any parent of a dysfluent child to enquire whether there is a speech therapist in their area who specializes in stammering. Such a therapist would have access to the most up-to-date information and treatment techniques for dysfluency.

Family therapy

Family therapists are usually psychologists, psychiatrists, social workers or other professionals who have been trained in how to help people who are having emotional problems. They have undertaken further training into how families function. People who work in this field look at a 'symptom' (such as bed-wetting, temper tantrums or withdrawal) in one family member, in terms of the whole family. Their intervention is therefore not with the person who has been identified as having the problem but with the family as a unit. They work not to change the individual or the symptom specifically but rather to change something about the way the family functions.

How family therapy is organized

Whilst there are many schools of family therapy, each with a slightly different approach, most therapists aim to see as many members of a family as possible, at least for some of the sessions. This is in order to gain an accurate picture of how the family functions.

Family therapists work in teams. One member conducts the interview while the others view the session from behind a one-way screen or on a simultaneously-transmitted video. While the therapist in the room speaks to the family, the rest of the team discuss what is happening and offer the therapist their views, either immediately through an earphone or in a face-to-face encounter during a break in the session. At the end of the session, the team produces some comments known as 'the intervention'. This is based on their understanding of how the family functions and may include ideas about change or a task for the family to carry out at home. The therapist does not take the side of any one individual but tries to understand the perspectives of all the family members. Sessions tend to take at least an hour and there is usually a two to four week gap between sessions. Families may receive up to ten or a dozen sessions of therapy: it is impossible to be more specific as both families and family therapists vary in their requirements.

Perhaps this way of working is easier to understand if we give some examples.

Michael, aged 14, has a stammer. Over the past few years it has become considerably worse. During this time, his parents have not been getting on so well. They communicate very little with each other. One of the few things they talk about is Michael's speech – they share a common concern in this area and when they are talking about it they do not quarrel. Perhaps Michael's stammer actually serves a function in keeping his parents together. If he no longer stammered they might have nothing to unite them.

Naheed is 5, the youngest of four children. He has recently started to stammer. His mother has always been at home with the children. If she gets a job, the whole family has fears that she may not be as available and they will have to face the unknown. Perhaps Naheed's stammer serves a function in keeping his mother available to the family. If he becomes more fluent and independent, his mother might feel more able to get a job.

It can seem that family therapists see families in a negative light. This is not the case. To the contrary, they believe that individual families function in the way they do because they are trying to maintain the family's stability, often in the face of enormous difficulties. Family therapy helps families understand what is going wrong and to draw on their strengths, improve their communication with each other, and identify ways of changing which will enable them to function more effectively to the benefit of all the members.

How to get a referral to family therapy

If you feel that your family may be helped by family therapy, you can refer yourself directly or ask another professional such as a speech and language therapist, family or hospital doctor or social worker to refer you. Young Minds Trust produced a leaflet in 1994 entitled *How Family Therapy can Help my Family* which, in addition to explaining the process of this kind of therapy, also helps people discover local services available. The Institute of Family Therapy have a leaflet *Information for Clients* which you may also find helpful. Both organizations can be found in the Useful addresses section.

Counselling

Counselling is currently undertaken by increasing numbers of speech and language therapists who have received further training in this area, or by professional counsellors. Counselling is really a form of structured listening. It is not advice-giving but rather a way of helping someone explore their difficulties and find their own solutions. Counsellors aim to create an atmosphere of trust in which clients feel able to talk over their problems, knowing they will be taken seriously and not judged. Counselling to help children who stammer is in two forms. Firstly there is the counselling of parents and carers. The purpose of this type of counselling is varied. Often it will be to help parents explore the ways in which they and others interact with their child, to discover those which are productive and those which are not so helpful. The counsellor tries to understand the feelings that parents have about the stammer and help them to reduce some of their negative emotions. We have already looked at how parents often feel guilty, embarrassed, angry and so on. Once these feelings have been identified, parents can be helped to view and respond to the stammer in a different way. Peter's father, for example, felt sorry for his son and would subconsciously try to save him from being hurt by talking for him. Counselling helped him to recognize what was happening, and he began to experiment with letting Peter talk for himself. He discovered that his son did not in fact stammer in all situations and even when he did, people were generally far more interested in what he had to say than in how he said it.

Counselling with parents of young children is likely to be preventive – to ensure that the child does not develop a negative self-image because of the speech dysfluency. Counselling for parents on occasions relates to other aspects of their lives. Perhaps one parent is experiencing some emotional difficulties which affect the way they interact with the child. Angela's mother, for example, was a great worrier and directed much of her concern towards her daughter. Counselling helped her look at and work to change other aspects of her life. Couple counselling helped Judith's parents take the decision to part. They had been staying together for the sake of Judith but the constant tension at home caused their daughter more distress than their eventual amicable separation.

Counselling is also used with children themselves. With younger children this does not necessarily occur through speech – play, drawing and music are also employed as a means of understanding how a child is feeling. As children get older, counselling generally becomes more verbal. Children are helped to express their feelings about stammering and experiment with ways of behaving, which allows them to view themselves more positively. All too often, stammering is seen as the only thing that matters. If a young person is to value other aspects of himself, such as sporting or academic achievements, aptitude, personality and so on, the effect of the stammer becomes less all-embracing. Counselling can also be useful for the young person who has habitually hidden his stammer, allowing him to become more open and hence freer in his communication with others. He may also come to realize that, although he seems unable to change the way he speaks, he does have a choice about how he feels and acts. Errol, for example, realized that he did not have to withdraw from speaking situations because he stammered. In fact he had as much right to express his views as anyone else. Although his stammer continued to be an inconvenience and upset him on occasions, he was generally more able to take control of his life, rather than let his stammer determine his actions.

It is often easier for children (and indeed adults) to talk freely to someone outside of the family. That person is not involved in their everyday life and will not be hurt in the way that parents may be, either by criticism of their behaviour or attitude or by hearing about the child's pain. This was highlighted to us recently when we asked a 15 year old with a severe stammer which had not reduced with therapy whether he wanted to continue attending or would prefer to have a break. He had no hesitation in choosing to continue – he told us that it made a big difference to him to be able to talk freely to someone who understood something about stammering. He knew we would empathize, not only about his difficulties but over his achievements. He felt these would seem trifling to others but were very important to him; for example, when he was able to ask for his own fare on the bus rather than request a friend to do it for him.

Information about counselling

The British Association for Counselling (BAC) have a number of publications which you might find helpful. On receipt of a stamped addressed envelope they will send you a list of counsellors and a leaflet *Counselling and Psychotherapy: Is it for me?* In addition they have a list of their publications for the general public. Their *Counselling and Psychotherapy Resources Directory* gives details of national organizations offering counselling, their local branches and lists of counsellors in private practice. If you are considering going for counselling, it is essential that you find out whether the counsellor adheres to a professional code of ethics. The BAC and Relate (Marriage Guidance) head office are in the Useful addresses section.

Self-help group: British Stammering Association

There is one main self-help organization currently operating nationally in Britain, The British Stammering Association. It is a registered charity based in London. The group consists of a number of salaried members, including a director. The rest of the work is carried out by volunteers and helpers, the majority of whom stammer themselves. The Association has a general committee who decide on policy and it also calls upon a number of specialist speech and language therapists who act as advisors.

At the time of its inception in 1978 the group's main concern was to support and provide information to adult stammerers. This has gradually changed and now the association believes it has an equally vital role to play with children who stammer and those involved in their care.

The British Stammering Association operates a helpline which anyone can call for advice, information and support. In addition it publishes a wide range of material including a quarterly magazine, advice leaflets for parents, teachers and others, and posters illustrating the difficulties stammering brings. Members also have access to a comprehensive library of books, audio and video materials relating to stammering.

Parents who contact the Association can expect a sympathetic response from someone who will have first-hand experience of the problems stammering creates. Parents can discuss their own personal difficulties and will receive advice and support, and may be referred for professional help to a local specialist speech and language therapist. The Association holds a directory of speech and language therapy services available for children across the country. An information pack is also provided to parents and adolescents who contact the Association. For parents of a younger child this pack contains details of the parents' network, the helpline, the Stammering Pupils Project network, information leaflets for parents and teachers, and information about the Association itself. The teenage pack includes leaflets specific to the age group (e.g. advice about talking on the telephone), a copy of the latest edition of the magazine *Speaking Out*, a list of useful books, audio and video material, and details of the Association. An information pack is also available for teachers.

The contact address and telephone number for the British Stammering Association is in the Useful addresses section.

Other sources of help

Books for children

We recently came across an article written in an American journal which reviewed a number of books written for children with a stammerer as a main character. Of the 20 books reviewed several were thought to represent stammering and the child who stammered in a realistic and helpful way, rather than just the nervous, anxious stereotype. We thought it would be useful to include details of these books here. Children who experience non-fluent speech often feel that they are the only ones with a talking problem and indeed there may be no one else in their class or school with a stammer. Being able to read about other children who feel the same and go through similar traumas can reduce the sense of isolation and may help the child feel better about their speech and themselves generally.

There may well be other books on the market which represent stammering but here we have only looked at a small selection which should be available from local libraries. We are sure that, whatever the age of the child or the difficulties he is experiencing, an adult wanting to find suitable and helpful reading material for the child will be well-advised to check the book(s) themselves to confirm the appropriateness of the content and any portrayal of stammering.

(1) *Emily Umily* by Kathy Corrigan. Published by Annick Press, Toronto, 1984. Suggested reading age: 4–7.

Emily is in reception class and her speech is quite dysfluent. She says 'um' a lot and other children in her class call her Umily and count the number of times she says 'um'. (Her dysfluency is not called stammering in the book.) Emily learns to see her 'ums' in a different light, reacts to them as acceptable sounds people make and her life becomes better as a result. Her speech does not appear to change.

(2) *Creole* by Stephen Cosgrove. Published by Price/Stern/Sloan, Los Angeles, 1983. Suggested reading age: 5–9.

Creole, a very ugly creature, meets a stammering alligator in the forest who does not run away from her unpleasant appearance. Creole then tells the alligator all the lovely things she wishes to say to the other forest creatures and the alligator repeats her words fluently to the animals. (The alligator only stammers when he speaks his own words.) The animals in the forest learn to like Creole as a result of how she helped the alligator speak. This book illustrates one feature of stammering speech: stammerers seem to have less difficulty speaking when using the same words as another person and speaking directly after them. Fortunately the author does not call this improvement in fluency in the alligator a cure, but the story is concluded satisfactorily.

(3) *Glue Fingers* by Matt Christopher. Published by Little, Brown and Company, Boston, 1975. Suggested reading age: 5–9.

Billy Joe stammers. He is so affected by his speech that he decides not to play football, which he loves, until his talking is better. Eventually he is persuaded to play and, despite his speech, he is accepted by the team.

(4) *Alan and the Animal Kingdom* by Isabelle Holland. Published by Lippincott, Philadelphia, 1977. Suggested reading age: 9–12.

Alan began stammering when he was 9, but is 12 in the story. Since starting to stammer he has learnt a number of ways of dealing with his speech, including keeping silent and rocking backwards and forwards when he speaks. Various characters in the book try and deal with Alan's speech: his teacher, his friends at school, all with varying degrees of success.

(5) *The Contrary Orphans* by Elizabeth Stucley. Published by Franklin Watts, New York, 1961. Suggested reading age: 9–15.

Two children are sent to an orphanage on the same day. Frankie Prust is one of the orphans and he has a bad stammer. In the course of the story Frankie comes to understand his speech difficulty and, with the help of a teacher, becomes more fluent.

(6) *The Skating Rink* by Mildred Lee. Published by Seabury Press, New York, 1969. Suggested reading level: 13–18.

Tuck Faraday is 15 and has a severe stammer. On his way home from school one day he meets Pete and the two become friends. Pete is very accepting of Tuck's speech and Tuck becomes more fluent as a result. Pete teaches Tuck how to skate and everyone is surprised by the results. Included in the story are some negative reactions to stammering: some characters think it is contagious, others believe Tuck is unstable. However, Tuck's own perceptions about his speech are central to the story and as he becomes less and less concerned about himself and more responsible for others, his speech seems less of a problem.

Other professionals

From time to time we see various other individuals and organizations offering to help people who suffer from stammering. They may advertise in national and local newspapers or magazines or indeed appear on the radio and television claiming to be able to help. Often they genuinely believe they have something to offer and perhaps have first-hand experience of the benefits in the methods they are offering to others. Occasionally their motives are less genuine. Some of these individuals may be hypnotherapists, some have a qualification in an aspect of medicine or psychology and usually operate in a private capacity.

While not wishing to dismiss these other possibilities of help out of hand, we would ask parents to take a cautious approach. In our experience stammering is a complex problem which requires careful handling by those who have considerable knowledge and expertise in the area.

When considering any type of help we suggest thinking about a number of issues:

- Is the person or organization registered in some way and secondly, are they registered with a professional body who has a code of ethics to which each member must adhere?
- Does the individual hold qualifications which are accredited by a professional body or institution?
- Is the individual or organization offering more than their own first-hand experiences?
- If the person or organization intends to see and offer your child some form of therapy are they (and you) covered by an insurance policy?
- Are you clear about what the person or organization is able to do for you and your child? Is there any evidence available that they can do what they claim? For example, can you talk to anyone who has undergone the same or similar treatment?
- Does the individual or organization have up-to-date knowledge about stammering in children or have they been offering the same approach for a number of years without modification?
- Is some form of follow-up programme offered after treatment?
- Does the British Stammering Association have any knowledge or experience of the programme or information the individual or organization is offering? (Does it check out?)

In this chapter we have tried to think about what we as parents look for when we are considering involving the help of others in our own difficulties. It is not an easy task to say what or who would help those whom we have never met! There is no one right answer or indeed perhaps no one right agency with all the answers for children who stammer. However, we hope that this section will have given you some idea of what is on offer at the moment, how different groups of people might help and which best meets your needs and those of the child who concerns you.

7

Stammering and school

Children spend a minimum of 11 years in school. They may attend for as many as 15 years. Inevitably these years are usually a mixture of good and bad times. If you look back to your own days at school you will probably, like us, have both happy and sad memories. At some times you will have felt good about your work, your friends and yourself, and other times you will have probably felt hopeless and helpless. The child who stammers also experiences the same variety of feelings as he grows and develops. In addition, however, he has the added difficulty of coping with his dysfluency – his own feelings about it and the reactions others have or he perceives them to have.

Schools have an enormous influence on the development of the child. Most parents want to ensure that their child's school years are happy and fruitful. In this chapter we will explore the ways in which parents with a child who stammers can help him cope most effectively and minimise any problems having a stammer may cause.

Choosing a school

Choosing is not an easy task. There are so many things to consider, not least the very practical issues of starting and finishing times, after-school provision, the location and the ease of journey. Sometimes these factors have to govern the choice we make – if we have no car and need to be at work for 9 a.m., it is no use sending a young child somewhere which entails a long bus ride. Assuming, however, that we do have some flexibility, what factors are important in considering a school for the child who stammers? We have chosen to look at schools for younger and for older age groups. The scope of this book does not allow us to look at all the educational and social factors parents need to think about in making their decision but rather those which are pertinent to dysfluency. Parents who would like more general information should contact the Advisory Centre for Education where they can purchase the book *School Choice and Appeal* (see Useful addresses).

Nursery and primary schools

There are many benefits for a child in some form of pre-school education. He learns to cope with change, to leave his parents for limited periods, to become accustomed to a structure and routine which increase when he starts school. He finds out about making choices and gains some independence skills. In meeting children of a similar age he inevitably finds out about the give and take of playing with others.

When considering a nursery or school it is very useful to visit and see the school in action. Most headteachers are only too happy to let parents come and look around before putting their child's name on the list. If they are not, we would be very suspicious! Hopefully parents will get a chance to meet the headteacher and a class teacher (although not necessarily the teacher the child will have) and even talk to pupils.

If the child can spend some time in the classroom, the child and the teacher get a chance to learn something about each other. The parent, too, finds out how the child feels about the experience, what he likes and does not like and what sort of preparation is likely to be most appropriate before he starts.

Points to explore

- Mention the child's dysfluency. See how the teachers react. Do they know much about the subject? Have they come across a dysfluent child before? If so, what was their experience? If not, do they have any preconceived ideas of what a dysfluent child is like? Are they interested to find out more?

- Find out how teachers might approach dysfluency. Would they expect the child to cope in exactly the same way as everyone else or make exceptions and treat the child very differently? (There can be difficulties in both these approaches as we will see later.) How does the teacher see the child – as a whole person or as a problem? Would she be prepared to alter class routines (such as registration) to accommodate the needs of the dysfluent child? Does the child have to ask for specific things: for example, to go to the toilet?

- Are the staff interested and prepared to listen to you and your ideas or concerns? Do they seem to encourage parental involvement?

- If your child is with you, observe how teachers interact with him. Do they address their remarks to you or are they keen to involve your child?

- Observe the children. Do they seem happy and relaxed? Is talking encouraged (within reason)? Are children generally given time and attention when they talk, are they listened to? Are their contributions welcomed?

- What is the teacher's attitude to the National Curriculum tests (SATs)? How are the tests managed? If the teacher appears anxious about the tests, is this attitude likely to rub off on the children and make them feel under pressure? How does the teacher prepare the children without raising anxieties?

- How easy is it to discuss difficulties which may occur? Does the school have an open door policy welcoming parents at any time or must an appointment be made?
- What are the school's policies on such areas as equal opportunities, discipline, punishment and bullying? Are they considered, well-written documents? Do they seem to be compatible with your own beliefs?
- Are there other children going to the school who your child already knows or who live in the neighbourhood and to whom they could be introduced before starting? (This may be more important for some children than for others.)
- What is the school's general attitude towards children with special needs – are they accepted and integrated into the school's routine or do they seem isolated in any way?

Secondary schools

Most secondary schools now organize open evenings for prospective new starters and their families. In our experience these usually involve a general talk followed by a visit around the school, and sometimes include the opportunity for an individual chat. If this latter is not available, it is a good idea to request such an appointment at an alternative time.

Points to explore

- The issue of friends is very important at this age and can be even more so for the dysfluent child. Few children are happy at 11 to go to a new school where they know no one. They have been at a stage in primary school where they have reached the top class and have a certain status. In the secondary school they may feel they are starting from the bottom rung of a long ladder. In addition, the dysfluent child often has a lot of security in the primary class where everyone knows him and accepts his stammer as just 'one of those things', in much the same way as they accept the child with glasses, a hearing aid, ginger hair and so on. In the secondary school he will be in different groups for different subjects and inevitably meet new people who know nothing about stammering. He may gain a lot of reassurance if there are children he knows and who understand him, who are at least in his registration group and whom he can meet at break times. A request to the school that he be placed in such a group will hopefully be met positively.

- The child may also feel reassured if he knows that there are or have been other children in the school who stammer and that staff have some experience of dealing with dysfluency. Obviously this cannot be manufactured but a quiet word to a teacher will ascertain the information.

- As with primary schools, it is important to find out how aware or interested the school are in the fact that the child stammers. Is it something they treat seriously and with concern? Do they want to find out how they can help – do they ask if the child is having therapy and suggest they get in contact? Are they willing to release the child for appointments and will they help to minimize any disruption this may cause?

- Are the teachers able to talk easily about stammering or do they seem awkward or embarrassed about it? Do you feel they will try to encourage the child to speak or are they more likely to collude with him in hiding the stammer?

- Is there a formal system of pastoral care? Are children encouraged to talk about difficulties they are experiencing and treated with respect when they do? Is information treated confidentially? Does the school have a counsellor and if so, how do children gain access?

- What sort of merit system does the school have? What is rewarded? Is it mainly academic success or does it include other aspects, such as behaviour, effort, attitude to others? Are children valued for what they are, not just for what they do?

- In the Personal and Social Education curriculum, is the discussion of personal issues and worries encouraged and are children helped to empathize with their peers?

- How does the school recognize and deal with teasing and bullying? Is there a written charter which all pupils sign and sanctions which are enforced if it is broken?

How to recognize and deal with problems at school

Sometimes, if we are lucky, our children tell us if they are having problems at school – that they have been teased, upset by someone's reaction, felt embarrassed, upset, worried about the way they have spoken. Sometimes (as we will see in the section on teasing) they may deny any difficulty but we will know that something is wrong by a change in their behaviour. However your child deals with their difficulties, it can be helpful if you suspect problems to contact the school and see if the cause can be identified and a solution found. Some typical problem areas in the classroom are dealt with below.

Reading

Many fluent children do not like reading out for a variety of reasons. They lack confidence in their ability, do not like to be the centre of attention or think they do not sound interesting. The child who stammers has the additional problem of not knowing if he will be fluent. He may fear (and be greeted by) laughter if he stammers. For the borderline or confirmed stammerer who changes words he anticipates having difficulty with, reading is often his greatest area of concern: the words are fixed and cannot be changed without others knowing. So how can teachers help?

- Perhaps the first point to make is that currently there seems to be less reading out in front of large groups than there used to be. Certainly, most primary school children do their reading practice in front of the teacher. If this is of concern to the child, it can help if the reading is done in a corner of the class where there is less likelihood of being overheard.
- It is also important to establish if the child has some problem with reading itself. If so, the dysfluency can occur as a response and extra help with reading may be required.
- With older children, it is often helpful to discuss problems individually. The aim should not be to single out the child with difficulties but rather to organize things differently to accommodate his needs. It is, for example, possible to arrange reading groups of three or four people in order to make the situation less threatening. Another possibility is, after discussion with the young person, to see if they would like prior warning of a reading session, so they have the opportunity to prepare their piece. For others, no waiting works best. Alternatively, some young people we know have an arrangement with their teacher so they can specify when they have their turn. This may mean that they always go first or last, for example, or they choose whether or not to read on a particular occasion. We generally do not think it is a good idea for children to be let off reading altogether. This all too often increases their feelings of difference or failure. However, there may be some occasions when reading out is creating so much worry for the child that a period of abstention is the only solution. In addition it can be helpful if children have a choice over whether to read out in very public events such as assemblies.

Registration

Giving a reply when your name is called on the register involves co-ordinating a number of factors. You need to concentrate closely in order to know when your name is coming; you often have to use a particular form of words ('Present', 'Yes, Miss Jones', 'Here' and so on); you must get the timing just right; and you are aware that for that split second the spotlight is on you. For the child who stammers this can present a number of difficulties. The actual words may be, or be perceived to be, difficult to say. Precise timing can be very hard when the slightest hesitation throws out the rhythm which has been established. Having all eyes and ears on you only increases the feeling of pressure.

This problem can be dealt with in a number of ways:

- The form of words required can be made less precise. Children can be told they can answer as they wish (within limits!). An imaginative teacher may even create interesting games around this activity – answer with the name of an animal, sport, how you are feeling, your favourite colour and so on. It is often easier if there is a number the child has to say rather than his name, although this is not always the case. Most teachers are prepared to be flexible if the problem is explained.
- Registration can be abandoned as a formal procedure, or the children may just be required to greet the teacher individually so that she can tick off their names.
- The register can be called when the children are moving around the classroom. This often takes off the pressure as others are not listening so intently.
- If it is not possible to persuade the teacher to alter the routine, it can be helpful to practise the form of words at home. This can be made fun: the child, for example, has to answer his parents in the name of the teacher. For example, when a parent calls the child or uses their name, he has to reply 'Yes, Mrs Shufflebottom'!

Oral participation It is not uncommon for dysfluent children, as they get older, to reduce their level of participation in order to hide the fact that they stammer. It is also not unusual for older children who do not stammer to do the same! This frequently makes it hard sometimes to be sure why the child is behaving in such a way. It is helpful to liaise with teachers to ascertain whether the child participates verbally and if the amount he says has reduced. Written reports should also make comments in this area. You will want to know if the child asks and answers questions. Will he argue his point or does he give up at the slightest difference of opinion? Does he ask his friends to voice his contributions for him? Does he say things in some lessons and not others? Is the size of the group a factor in whether he speaks? Is he more prepared to talk to one person than in front of the whole class? Does he frequently say he doesn't know an answer when the teacher feels this is not the case? Is there a big difference between his oral and written contributions?

When it comes to formal presentations, plays and so on, it is important that assumptions are not made as to whether the child should or wants to take part. The situation should be discussed with the child so that he is given some choice in the decision taken.

We would want to encourage children to participate in class in a way which is not related to the level of fluency. In other words we would wish them to feel able to express their opinions, tell their news, ask for clarificaton where necessary and reply to questions when they know the answer.

Foreign language lessons

These can pose a particular problem for the child who stammers, especially as, certainly initially, they are often almost exclusively oral. Unlike some other lessons where participation is encouraged but not essential, in language lessons every child is usually expected to take part verbally. Sometimes the introduction of a second language occurs when the child is also coping with settling into a new school. If your child seems to be having some difficulty in these lessons it is first necessary to establish why. Is it, in fact, because he is finding the language itself difficult or is it connected with the stammer? If it is the latter, then what can be done? Talking to your child is a good starting point. What does he see as the problem? Does he, for example, find he is more likely to stammer because the words are less easy to pronounce, is it the reaction of others when he stammers which troubles him, or is it the fact that he has to say a particular form of words and is not able to use his avoidance strategies? Once the problem is identified there are a number of ways in which it can be approached. A discussion with the teacher should help to ascertain possible ways forward. If the language itself is a problem, extra help can be given or perhaps the child may need to be placed in a set in which he feels more able to cope. If it is the reactions of others to the stammer, then this will need sensitive handling. Ideas can be taken from the section of this chapter which deals with teasing. Should the difficulty occur because the child cannot avoid words, this area of concern can be tackled in a variety of ways, such as helping the child look at how to cope with adverse reactions which he feels could result, assisting him to reduce his word avoidance (probably in conjunction with a speech and language therapist), discussing with the teacher when the child finds it easier to talk (in a small group, at the beginning, middle or end of the lesson and so on) and, if appropriate, talking to the class about his difficulties and enlisting their support.

One final point needs to be made in this section. Many dysfluent children do *not* find foreign language lessons a particular problem, so it is important we do not anticipate a difficulty that will not be apparent. Indeed, some children may find they cope better in these lessons than in others; perhaps just because they are good at the subject or even because when they are 'playing the role' of a foreign speaker, they find talking easier.

Other problem areas in school

Subject choices

Around the age of 14, most children have to make choices as to which subjects they will study to at least GCSE level and which they will drop. This can be a difficult choice for any child to make, but the child who stammers is sometimes influenced by his dysfluency. There may be a temptation to let the decision be over-affected, not by personal preference or past academic performance, but by the amount of oral contribution required. It is important, therefore, to try to find out the basis for the decisions your child makes. If you feel that the stammer has been an influential factor, the situation should be discussed with the child and with relevant teachers to see if there are ways in which it could be modified to make other options possible. Let us take the example of Kathy who both likes and is good at French, but fears the oral component. She decides to take an alternative subject which she enjoys less and at which she is not so good academically. There may be a number of alternatives which might make Kathy reconsider her decision. By discussing her oral contribution with the teacher, ways could be found to lessen any pressure she feels – the teacher may talk to the class about her difficulties if appropriate, oral work could be done in small groups, and warning given of formal oral assessments – which it might even be possible to arrange on a one-to-one basis. In addition, Kathy can be told that a letter can be sent to the examination board, explaining that she has a stammer so that allowances will be made for any lack of fluency which occurs.

The playground and dining hall

Although the teacher usually has a good idea about how the child is coping in the classroom situation, the playground and dining halls are areas in which he is less frequently observed. Casual enquiries as to how the child spent his mealtimes and who he was with can help a parent ascertain if there are any problems. If parents suspect that the child is either spending long periods alone or is being teased in the playground or is having difficulty in asking for his meal, it is a good idea to contact the school to see if any more can be found out. A dinner lady or teacher on duty may be able to observe the child and assess the situation. If there does appear to be a problem, then it should be explored with the teacher and child.

Time off for speech and language therapy appointments

Many children who attend for therapy are quite happy for their peers to know and do not mind leaving school even in the middle of a lesson if necessary. We are always glad to know this is the case and that the child is open about his stammer and his therapy. Some children, however, find this quite a problem. They are not prepared to mention their stammer to others or to let their classmates know they attend for therapy. While we do not want to collude with hiding the stammer, neither do we want to increase the child's feelings of difference. We would try, therefore, to ensure that the child attends at a time which causes him the least possible distress. Another important consideration in the timing of appointments is the amount of school work missed. Whilst it is not always possible to offer appointments out of school time, nor for reasons of timetabling to offer an appointment at a different time each week, most therapists would try to be as flexible as possible and to bear the following points in mind:

- the child should miss as little school as possible;
- lessons missed should be those which all involved consider to be the ones from which the child can most afford to be absent or on which he can catch up most easily;
- the child should be able to leave and return to school at a time which causes him the least possible upheaval or concern.

If the child is adamant that he does not want others to know where he is going, we would suggest the teacher respects the child's feelings. It may be useful for child or parent to discuss this with the teacher and formulate a possible response to enquiries from other children regarding the child's absences from school.

On occasions, the problems the child incurs in attending for speech and language therapy, in terms of missed lessons or teasing, outweigh the benefits. In such cases, therapy may, at least temporarily, have to be at arms' length – perhaps individual or group therapy in the holiday periods, and work with parents or teachers to help them to modify the effects of the problems the stammer is causing.

Talking about stammering

We have already mentioned that we feel it is preferable for children to be open about their stammering rather than pretend it does not exist or try at all costs to conceal it. Such courses of action usually only worsen the problem in the long term by making the child feel guilty, embarrassed or ashamed of themselves, and use all manner of tricks and devices to avoid stammering.

Sometimes, with encouragement, children can be helped to talk more openly about their stammering and thus to see it more as something they *do* rather than something they *are*. We have found the following useful in this process:

- Conversations with the child and appropriate teacher(s) in which stammering is discussed sensitively, problems raised and solutions explored.
- Ensuring that all teachers are aware of the child's speech problem. If this is the case, they are less likely to be taken aback if stammering occurs. They should be given ideas as to how to respond, which reactions help and which hinder, and how to encourage oral participation. The leaflet *The Child who Stammers: A Guide for Teachers* offers excellent ideas. It is available for a nominal fee through the British Stammering Association (see the Useful addresses section).
- Discussion in the classroom about problem areas. This can happen in a variety of ways. It may be very general. As children with special needs are being integrated more and more into mainstream schools, children are becoming increasingly aware of the needs of those with sensory deprivations (for example, sight or hearing loss), mobility problems (for example, children with special shoes or in wheelchairs) or with learning difficulties. More emphasis is put on children as individuals and on respecting and understanding those with particular needs. Discussions of a general nature can therefore have a knock-on effect on children who stammer. Discussions may also be more specific to speech. The teacher could talk about the importance of listening to others, waiting if someone is having difficulty in saying

what he wants to for whatever reason (for example, nervousness, forgetting the word, not being sure of the answer or even stammering). On occasions it can be helpful to talk about the specific child. Usually this would be with the child's permission. It may or may not involve the child directly.

- Sometimes children are asked to give talks on a subject of their choice. We know of several who have chosen to talk about stammering in such a forum. These have generally been very positive experiences. The child has been surprised at how interested others are, at the number of questions raised at the end of the talk and the increased understanding.

- We have given talks about stammering at secondary schools, either in a year or part-year assembly or in a Personal and Social Education lesson, when a young person has felt this would be useful. In our presentations we first explain a little about the nature of stammering. We then show a short clip from the video *A Voice in Exile* (available on loan from the British Stammering Association). In this a young man stammers in school and is laughed at. We invite the children to consider how this might make him feel and we are always impressed by the quality of the answers and the empathy shown by the young people. We go on to invite them to explore appropriate and inappropriate responses to people who stammer. Our young clients tell us that their peers' understanding of their difficulties has increased as a result and generally they then find it easier to talk about stammering with them.

Teasing and bullying

This is an area which schools currently take very seriously. Many now have a 'bullying charter' which all pupils have to sign, and transgressions are regarded as very serious matters.

It is not always easy to know if a child is being teased or bullied. Some children wear their hearts on their sleeves and do talk about such things very easily. Some are extremely sensitive and become upset over what may in fact have been a throw-away remark which was not meant to cause offence. Others say nothing about responses which trouble them but instead bottle up their feelings. Sometimes the cork on the emotional bottle pops and the child reacts in an inappropriate way or at an inappropriate time. In other children the cork just comes out a little at a time – the child changes his behaviour, becomes moody, awkward, sullen, shy and so on.

There is no magic formula for finding out if a child is being teased. However, if the home environment is one in which people are encouraged to talk over difficulties and discuss solutions calmly and rationally, the child *may* feel it is safe to talk about such things. In addition, if a child's behaviour changes and a parent suspects that all is not well, an appropriate careful enquiry is sometimes all that is needed for the child to spill the beans.

If a child tells a parent that he is being teased or bullied, what should be done? Once again there is no easy answer and any solution will depend in part on the following questions:

- How big is the problem? Are we talking about a one-off situation or something which occurs more often?
- What was the intention behind it? Were the remarks intended to hurt or were they just interpreted as hurtful? A child may, for example, ask 'Why do you talk like that?' and want to know exactly that. Alternatively, the question may indeed have been asked in order to humiliate.
- How many people are involved? Is it just one person or are there a group of people either doing the teasing or being teased?
- Is the teasing specific to stammering or is it about something else altogether? It is easy to jump to conclusions if we feel sensitive about something.
- Does he bully others? Is the bullying he receives a reaction to that?

Having ascertained something about the nature of the teasing, what might happen next? There are a number of possibilities as to how parents may act:

- It could be that all that is needed is discussion of the incident with the child, perhaps to look at how and why it occurred and then help the child to feel differently about either the situation or himself. John, for example, tells his parents that his best friend Mark laughed when he stammered in reply to a question from the teacher. It may be that, in discussing the situation with his parents, John discovers that Mark was actually laughing about his answer rather than his stammer.
- Another way of dealing with teasing is to try to boost the child's confidence. All children are likely to be teased at some point in their school career, and it is important that they learn to toughen themselves enough to tolerate a certain amount which is not intended to be malicious. If a child's self-esteem is good, he is likely to be able to cope better. Let us look at an example. When Billy goes into a shop to ask for sweets, he stammers and another child mimics him. Billy is a confident child and tells himself that it is the other child who is at fault.

While the mimicking naturally hurts somewhat, it doesn't affect him unduly or for too long.

Parents have an important role in developing their children's self esteem. Children need to feel valued for what they are, not for what others might want them to be. They require recognition and praise for their achievements and support when things do not go as well as they had hoped. Consistent and fair discipline provides boundaries and security (as discussed in Chapter 5). Self-esteem is an important factor in the child's development. The child who stammers may have to be given extra support in order that the dysfluency does not negatively affect his growing sense of self. He must be able to separate the way he talks from the way he is, so they do not become enmeshed. He needs to know that his parents' regard for him is unconditional, that it does not vary according to his speech. If, for example, he perceives that his parents seem embarrassed if he stammers in front of their friends, or even speak for him rather than let them see him stammer, he can come to feel they value him less because he stammers. He may learn to feel the same about himself as a consequence.

Parents can also help by arming their child with more effective strategies to cope with teasing. Very often, children stick to one or two strategies which are not always helpful. Stuart, for example, tells the boys who tease him to 'shut up' – and they continue all the more. Kevin has been known to hit out and then ends up getting into trouble himself. There is no one effective way which works for all teasers or all who are teased, but the following are ideas which are helpful in some cases:

- 'Ignore' the stammering. This is more easily said than done! However, it is very effective. The object of teasing is to get a reaction – if none comes, the teaser will usually give up in time. A boy of 14 whom we knew told us 'When they laugh at me, I tell myself that it is they who have the problem and then I don't mind nearly as much'.
- Acknowledge and accept the remarks made by the offender. This is a strategy that some older children find useful. A response such as 'Yes, I do have a stammer' can take the wind out of the sails of someone who is aiming for a different sort of response. In addition, some children find they can make a remark which stops the teasing progressing. If, for example, a child is mimicked in a particular way, he might correct the mimicker and say something along the lines of 'Well, at least get it right, I said 'M . .M . .M . .M . .Monday' not 'Mu . . Mu . . Monday'.
- Laugh at the stammer yourself. Sometimes this takes the sting out of

the situation. However, if done too often it may make others take the stammer superficially and the hurt that teasing can cause is never seen. The child who stammers could then feel unable to react in any other way.

- Sometimes it is necessary to encourage the child to tell a teacher about the teasing or even inform the teacher yourself. This could be the case if the teasing is more severe or ongoing and the child is unable or unwilling to use appropriate strategies, or if the strategies used do not produce the desired effect. Children are often loath to talk to teachers, fearing that doing so will make the situation worse – they will not only be teased but also identified as someone who 'tells' on others. In our experience, however, teachers usually deal with such situations very sensitively. Sometimes the offender is unaware of the upset he is causing; he thinks of it merely as harmless fun. If the reality is pointed out he often feels ashamed and ceases what he is doing. On occasions a more forceful reaction is needed, such as a sharp word or reminder of what will happen if the offence continues – apologies to be made, detentions, the headmaster seen, extra homework or even in some cases, suspension.

- Parents can provide a forum for the child to express his feelings in a variety of ways. Some children find it helpful if this is physical – punching cushions, banging a drum, having a good shout, playing football or going for a run. Drawing or writing stories about bullying can be useful. There are also several books written for children on this subject (some are listed in Chapter 6). Sometimes it helps to 'act out' feelings; the child, for example, pretends that an empty chair is actually the bully and tells him in no uncertain terms exactly what he thinks of him.

Summary

In this chapter we have looked at problems that stammering may cause in schools and how best to manage them. Although we have discussed a number of areas which give rise to concern, we feel it is important to stress that many children who stammer cope extremely well in the school environment and feel supported and encouraged by peers and teachers alike. If parents are aware of possible areas of concern, look for warning signs and establish a dialogue with their children and the teachers, many of these problems can be effectively reduced or even avoided.

8

Final thoughts

Collectively we have worked with people who stammer for over 30 years. We are frequently amazed at how much enjoyment and satisfaction we continue to get out of our work, even after all this time. One reason may be that the area in which we both specialize is so diverse and varied. We cannot predict with any certainty who will walk into our clinic next, how their dysfluent speech will present itself or affect their lives. This means that we are constantly challenged and stimulated by new problems and difficulties. Boredom and routine are certainly not things which appear in our job descriptions!

However, it is due to this lack of predictability that we continue to learn about stammering and non-fluency in children even now. We do not believe we have all the answers, and so consideration of some final thoughts is rather difficult under these circumstances. Our own ideas are still evolving and changing. Indeed the type of therapy we offer to children currently is quite different from that which we carried out only five years ago. We are not ashamed of this change. Indeed, we believe that when we stop learning from our clients, from research and from experience, that will be the time to quit.

So rather than try to summarize some aspects of stammering or approaches to the difficulties associated with it (which we may have a different perspective on next year), in this final section we will instead outline developments that we would like to see in the future.

Research

As we have said earlier in this book, much of the information we have from scientific studies is at best unclear and at worst contradictory. We desperately need several researchers to look at lots of children in order to find out exactly how dysfluency develops and, perhaps more importantly, to establish what keeps it going in each child's case. In the 1970s a survey of speech problems was carried out in Newcastle-upon-Tyne. This produced some very valuable information which is still used today. However, as we know so much more now and have better and more sophisticated computer packages, a similar study carried out in the 1990s would yield a lot more information and indeed be a giant leap forward for stammering.

It would be nice to know the cause of stammering, but to be realistic it seems probable that there is no one simple answer. The signs seem to point to several factors contributing to its occurrence. So perhaps researchers should continue to keep their options open and look at all possibilities. It may be at the end of the day that we discover one causal factor for one group of people and another for another group. For example, genetic factors may be important where the dysfluency is of a particular type, and rate of speaking may be crucial with a group of children who have poor control over their muscles. At the moment none of these links have been made and so information must continue to be gathered.

Of course it would be wonderful if a cure could be found. We would be among the first to shake the discoverer by the hand and hang up our therapy hats. Once again the portents suggest that this is some way off. It seems likely that a cure will be the 'chicken' that follows when the causation 'egg' has been cracked. But we must not be despondent. As far as children are concerned we know that the recovery rate is increasing, the number that go on to stammer in adult life is falling, so we must be doing something right!

Society's attitude to stammering

While we beaver away in our own clinics we are aware of greater difficulties in the outside world which affect the people we see. The way society reacts to stammerers whether they are children or adults is something which concerns us greatly.

Firstly, there is the 'say nothing' approach, which we have discussed at some length. This is appropriate when the child is happily non-fluent and unaware of anything wrong with his talking. However, when a child is obviously distressed and worried then his need for support and concern should be met.

So often we have heard sad tales from adults who longed to be able to discuss their anxieties with a caring adult. Admittedly the adult may not have been able to do anything constructive, but these clients describe a desire just to have been able to share their problems and receive comfort and reassurance. It is our belief that society needs to develop a more open attitude to this speech difficulty in the way that it is beginning to have in other areas such as physical disability, Aids-related illnesses and abuse of children.

Secondly, there is the presumption about what stammering actually is and means for the person who stammers. We are tired of the stereotyped stammerer portrayed in the media: the nervous, anxious individual, repressed and with a hint of 'not quite the full shilling'. We meet this attitude too when we tell people what type of work we do. There is often a genuine interest in stammering and people are frequently keen to know all there is to know – but then the old chestnut appears 'Why do they do it then? Is it because they are nervous?' In many ways it is hardly surprising that the general population arrive at this conclusion since most likely they will experience some degree of non-fluent speech when they themselves are nervous about a speaking situation. Nevertheless, the time has come for a change and people need to be educated. Schools need to play their part in developing a more understanding attitude, and perhaps more information could be given to both teachers and GPs in training to prepare them for their role in managing stammering. If as a society we have a greater understanding of ethnic minorities, of the role of women, of disabilities in general, then surely we can apply the same principles to a small group of the population who happen to speak a little differently. Let us start to treat them as individuals rather than stereotypes.

Access to help

Our final thought is about being able to get help. Once again our experience with parents and adult clients we see is that getting to the clinic is a battle in itself. We hear reports of parents who have recognized their child's difficulties from quite an early age and sought help unsuccessfully. They may have discussed it with their health visitor, GP or other professional but not managed to secure an expert opinion. Very often they struggle on, try to read the right books or even visit a hypnotherapist to see if that works. The big stumbling block is that many people, including some in the medical profession, believe stammering is something children will grow out of by themselves. Well, of course they are half right. Many children, as we have discussed in Chapter 2, do indeed experience normal non-fluent speech and then go on to talk without difficulty. However, that period of normal non-fluency has to be handled correctly and the child must feel confident about their talking irrespective of the fluency problems. Parents and other carers need to know how to help the child through this crucial period and, as speech and language therapists, we believe we have a role to play in this. We would reemphasize at this point that speech and language therapists operate an open referral system and any parent or carer who is concerned about a child's speech can refer to us directly. It is important that therapists see children who are experiencing some non-fluency as soon as anyone is concerned. We believe we can help.

We are aware, however, that not all areas have speech and language therapy provision for dysfluent children. This is a situation that is cause for much concern. It makes no sense to defer treatment or hope that the problem will just go away. If these children do not receive help at the very time when it is most needed then the problem experienced by individuals will often be greater and ultimately may well pose a greater burden on the health service as they struggle with the dysfluency as adults.

Not only does the complete lack of provision in some places give cause for concern, but the absence of therapists specializing in the field is also worrying. We know from our contact with other colleagues that many of them have a specific interest in stammering and would appreciate the opportunity to specialize. However, not every provider of health care employs a specialist in this field and certainly the number of full-time posts is limited to a handful. It is our belief that the nature of the work with dysfluent children and adults is such it requires a therapist specializing in dysfluency to do it justice. We are indebted to our friends in the British Stammering Association who help bring these issues to the attention of Health Authorities and local populations. However, there is a need for others to let their voices be heard. In Britain all dysfluent children should have access to a local specialist service, but even this is not enough. We think there should be a number of centres of excellence scattered around the country offering special treatment and facilities to these individuals within the NHS.

Conclusion

Our final words are specifically to the children themselves and their parents. We are all too familiar with what a devastating problem stammering can be. We have seen children who could not say a single word without the most enormous struggle and whose lives were limited by the fear of how other people would respond to their speech difficulties. However, we have also seen them change. Some of them have learnt to control their speech and, perhaps more importantly, to manage the fear and other feelings that accompanied the speech problem. Their parents have been able to move on too, to hear what their child was saying and not focus on the stammering speech all the time.

One particular child comes to mind at this point. Stuart had one of the worst stammers we had heard or seen. It happened on almost every word and was accompanied by lots of distracting sounds, facial expressions and little body movements which were his attempts at forcing the words out of his mouth. From our perspective his stammer was incredibly resistant – it defied our best efforts. We tried to reduce its frequency and severity using all the techniques in our armoury. In the end it was marginally better: it still occurred as often but with less of the struggling behaviours. Crucially, however, Stuart reached the stage of being able to accept it and move on. He went to University, pursued his chosen career and even took up amateur dramatics. We do not think we would have predicted such an outcome, but it illustrated for us that even the severest stammer does not have to be one which stops a child saying what he wants to say, doing what he wants to do and being the person he is inside.

Useful addresses

British Stammering Association
15 Old Ford Road
Bethnal Green
London E2 9PJ
Tel. 0181 983 1003
Helpline: 0181 981 8818

British Association for Counselling
1 Regent Place
Rugby
Warwickshire CV21 2PJ
Tel. 01788 578 328/9

Royal College of Speech and Language Therapists
7 Bath Place
Rivington Street
London EC2A 3DR
Tel. 0171 613 3855

Institute of Family Therapy
43 New Cavendish Street
London WIM 7RG
Tel. 0171 935 1651

Relate (Marriage Guidance)
Herbert Gray College
Little Church Street
Rugby
Warwickshire
Tel. 01788 573241

Young Minds Information Service
22a Boston Place
London NW1 6ER
Tel. 0171 724 7262

Advisory Centre for Education
1B Aberdeen Studios
22 Highbury Grove
London N5 2EA
Tel. 0171 354 8321

Further reading

The British Association for Counselling (BAC), 'Counselling and Psychotherapy: Is it for me?' (leaflet), (BAC), 4th edition, 1994.

Christopher, Matt, *Glue Fingers*, Little, Brown and Company, Boston, 1975.

Corrigan, Kathy, *Emily Umily*, Annick Press, Toronto, 1984.

Cosgrove, Stephen, *Creole*, Price/Stern/Sloan, Los Angeles, 1983.

Goffe, Toni, *Bully for You*, Playring Ltd, 1991.

Holland, Isabelle, *Alan and the Animal Kingdom*, Lippincott, Philadelphia, 1977.

The Institute of Family Therapy (IFT), 'Information for Clients' (leaflet), IFT, 1995.

Lawson, Sarah, *Helping Children Cope with Bullying*, Sheldon Press, 1994.

Lee, Mildred, *The Skating Rink*, Seabury Press, New York, 1969.

Peters, T J, and Guitar, B, *Stuttering: An integrated approach to its nature and treatment*, Williams & Wilkins, Baltimore, 1991.

Sheehan, J G, and Martyn, M M, 'Spontaneous Recovery from Stuttering', *Journal of Speech and Hearing Research*, 9, pages 121–35, 1966.

Stones, Rosemary, *Don't Pick on Me*, Piccadilly Press, 1993.

Stucley, Elizabeth, *The Contrary Orphans*, Franklin Watts, New York, 1961.

Young Minds Trust (YMT), 'How Family Therapy can Help my Family' (leaflet), YMT, 1994.

Index